Turning Back
the
Hands of Time

Turning Back
the
Hands of Time

Dr. John Emmett

Abecedarian Books
Baltimore, Maryland

TURNING BACK THE HANDS OF TIME

Library of Congress
Cataloging-in-Publication Data
ISBN 0-9763106-0-0

Library of Congress Card Catalog Number:
2004115874

Second Printing

For more information, please refer to our website:
www.nufitness.net

Published by

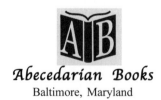

Abecedarian Books
Baltimore, Maryland

Manufactured in the United States of America

Dedication

I dedicate this book to my wife Margie, the most beautiful woman on earth, and to my two little scholar athletes, Alexis and John.

Margie, I dedicate this book to you because of your patience, strength, and enduring love. Also, thanks for your ability to impeccably manage all the madness, which I impart upon our life.

And lastly to my children, please don't forget what daddy tells you are the most important things in life: God, family, education, and sports. Listen to your mother, and do what she says. I love you all.

Contents

FOREWORD

THE ART & SCIENCE OF PHYSICAL CHANGE

You hold in your hands a blueprint for physical change, *true* physical change—not imagined changes or miniscule changes, not inconsequential changes or barely noticeable changes— significant, measurable, *irrefutable* changes. If you are desirous and determined to change the current condition of your body, if you are serious about positively altering the composition of your physique and health, then read on: you have a manual that will provide you a game plan and a map for where you want to go. In this age of fakesters, hucksters, and outright fitness frauds, Dr. John Emmett is the real deal—a rare individual, a medical professional, and a champion bodybuilder. John not only can talk the talk, he walks the walk. I could not think of a better mentor or guide for people who are serious about altering their body for the better. In this day and age, fitness experts seem to break down into two broad categories: those who pontificate about change but do so from a theoretical vantage point, and those who rely on street smarts, gym rats that have built bodies that border on surreal but preach methods that have no relevance for normal folks who work serious jobs, have families, responsibilities, and commitments. There are few fitness experts who combine the best theoretical knowledge science and modern medicine have to offer with real world empirical gym knowledge and genuine athletic exploits.

Dr. John Emmett is such a man—a surgeon and a champion bodybuilder who has built a physique that has to be seen to be believed. Yet he has a real life: wife, kids, commitments galore, a thriving surgical practice and enough energy to power Three Mile Island. Who better to consult about renovating your physique and health? Anyone dissatisfied with the status of their current physical condition would be well advised to take a long careful read of this book.

In a way it's a deceptive opus. Dr. John has a folksy quality in his writing that makes you feel as if he is in the room with you, the two of you talking as old friends might about a subject they are passionate about. Between the pages of this book are some of the best scientific explanations about how and why the human body reacts in certain ways to certain procedures: why certain foods, exercise regimens, and modes elicit certain results. John weaves together a comprehensive eating and training regimen and provides a fitness schematic, a game plan, a methodology immediately applicable to the particulars of your situation. Modern life is hectic and demanding and the biggest complaint I hear from folks wanting to get serious about fitness is that they don't have the time. Time management is one of Dr. Emmett's specialties. He can show you how to weave fitness into the complex fabric of modern life.

His methods are sound, tried and proven: eat hearty, eat often but eat 'clean.' Exercise need not be time intensive but it need be intense. Old school traits like perseverance, discipline, tenacity, and patience are integral to the John Emmett approach to body renovation. If you follow his approach and do so for a protracted period of time, success, by any measure, is a foregone conclusion. Dr. John can supply the plan if you can supply the tenacity. His approach requires intense weight and cardioexercise. Workouts are strung together like pearls on a strand: day by day, week by week. Consistent application reaps huge cumulative results. He believes diet/nutrition to be upwards of 80% of fitness success –

a pronouncement that has huge implications. He shows the patient reader how to construct an eating plan that will ensure a complete physical makeover. Exercise, combined with his approach to eating, results in amazing changes in very short order. He has demonstrated this repeatedly in himself and in those around him who seek his council. For those who are serious and apply John's approach, physical renovation lies just around the corner.

It really all comes down to you, dear reader; if you *burn* for physical change then you've found the source—Dr. John Emmett. He will never tell you that the path is easy, but he can show you the way. He knows the way because he's blazed the path himself. He's not pontificating to you; he's sharing with you the methods, modes and philosophies that have made him a champion and allowed him to sculpt a physique Michelangelo would have deemed perfection-made-flesh. John didn't achieve his physical success in a vacuum: he's a 43-year old surgeon with two kids, a mortgage payment and like you he deals with all the hassles and tribulations modern life throws in our path – yet he makes it work and he can show you how to make it all work. He can make fitness and physical renovation work for you if you'll let him. John is never one to make braggadocios pronouncements or outrageous claims…he's just a guy who successfully built one of the best physiques in the country for a man over forty, this despite living life to its fullest – John Emmett can do the same for you if you give him half a chance….

John Parrillo
2004

ACKNOWLEDGMENTS

First and foremost, I would like to acknowledge Mr. John Parrillo and his lovely wife, Dominique. Without Mr. Parrillo, none of this would have been possible. Thousands of athletes around the world, including myself, who follow Mr. Parrillo's principles are stronger and leaner because of his fitness and nutrition philosophies. Make no mistake, the words in my book convey John Parrillo's philosophy and trust me when I say I have not even scratched the surface. I highly recommend you gather all the information he has to offer for a stronger, leaner, and healthier lifestyle.

Dr. Cliff Sheats is the most brilliant nutritionist I've ever had the pleasure of knowing. Dr. Cliff Sheats and Mr. Parrillo pioneered the high calorie nutritional program for fat loss years ago. Dr. Sheats is the author of *Lean Bodies* and the founder of the Lean Bodies nutritional program. Thank you for all you have taught me.

Mr. Marty Gallagher is simply the best fitness writer in the business. He currently writes for the *Washington Post,* and I'd like to thank him for all the work he's done for me over the years. When I don't know how to express the words, you are always there to help make me sound brilliant. Thank you.

Mr. Tim Rogers and TWR Photography. Thank you so much for your professional, artistic, and amazing photographic capabilities.

Ms. Celeste Chance, your artistic style and professionalism with body color is simply unbelievable.

Ms. Lizzie Nimmich and Patrick Klein, thank you so much for your hard work in reading my chicken scratch, which I called my book, and transcribing it to disk form so it could actually be edited.

Mr. Peter Hyerman and Bear Press, thank you for your hard work in editing the original manuscript.

Ms. Diane Hernandez, Esquire, thank you so much for proofreading the final manuscript of my book. Your insight is marvelous and you're a wonderful sister-in-law. I love you.

To Mr. Richard Meltzer, founder of The Digital Planet, thank you so much for the superb job in graphic design for the front and back cover of this book.

To the best friends I have, Mr. Bruce Brooks and his wife Yvette Hernandez-Brooks, Mr. David Bender, Mr. David Levine and his wife Ellen, and Mr. Ron Green and his wife Gail. Thank you all for allowing me to use your names and stories in the book. The friendships that Margie and I have developed with you make our lives complete.

To my mother, father, sister, and in-laws, thank you all so very much for believing in me and giving me the family support to pursue projects like this. To Mom and Dad, I love you so much, thanks for giving me the opportunity to become a successful surgeon. And a special thank you to Mom for proofreading the original manuscript.

Chapter I

"You're Going To Eat More Food..."

To the newcomer, *Turning Back the Hands of Time* is a guidebook for achieving the physique of your dreams; to you who are familiar with my methods, it is a sourcebook for answers to any questions you might have. In these pages you will find a system of nutrition and exercise that can permanently replace all fad diets and failed exercise regimens. Here is something that works. Now get ready to eat more food than you've ever eaten in your entire life!

It's not as easy as it sounds. I can't make these changes for you. Only you can do that. You allow me to give you the knowledge, but you must find it in yourself to get it done.

This is a journey away from the complexities of the myriad modern diets and fitness methods into a world where your eating and exercise habits are governed by a simple principle: your own goals. If what you want is a healthy body, but you don't want to eat like a parakeet, then *Turning Back the Hands of Time* can get you there. With the aim of achieving a lean, healthy physique, this book defines the exercise technique and nutritional balance you need to get there. The physique of your dreams can be achieved. Whether you want to take off fifty pounds of fat—permanently—or decrease your body fat composition to 4% or 5%, step on stage and compete in your first bodybuilding competition, it can be done. If you aren't disabled or the victim of life-threatening illness, it can be done. Whether you are twenty-two or seventy-five, it can be done. Whether you are male, female, athletic, or a couch potato, it can be done. All you need is enough self-discipline to get going.

The good thing is I've done a lot of the work for you. After years of feasting, fasting, training, competing, and reading everything under the sun, I've made the most of my mistakes, and learned from them. I know the pitfalls and the toeholds. With that knowledge I'll help you find your way to *Turning Back the Hands of Time*.

Sound exciting? It is, but it's not easy. It's like your parents told you: good things come to those who try. This journey is hard, but it's hardly impossible. I have done it, and so have many others. Like any difficult road it has its rewards, and these will outweigh the obstacles. The first thing to understand is that this journey can empower you to be what you want to be for many years to come. You are embarking on an entirely new life style. The main goal here isn't to take off ten pounds in a week. This is the way for you to turn your life around and head in a newer, younger direction: it's the long run and the real deal. And, as I said before: Get ready to eat more food than you've ever eaten in your entire life!

This book is for those of you who have tried time and time again to get in shape. It is aimed at anyone who has made the effort through diet, exercise or both. If you have spent outlandish amounts of money on exercise equipment that simply didn't work, or peeled off pounds on a quick-loss diet, only to see them return, you may be ready. If you find yourself looking at every diet ad and every health club commercial, this may be the book for you. If you have reached the end of your rope and will do just about anything to finally change your life and reach your personal goals, then I think I can help. Do any of these descriptions fit you? Then follow me. I will teach you what to do, when to do it, and you will finally get it done! And you will keep on getting it done because this is not another ten-day or two-week diet. If you need to drop forty pounds and be svelte and beautiful in two weeks time, consult your nearest supermarket tabloid.

A program that works won't make those promises. A truly workable regimen requires focus, discipline, and consistency. So, I ask: Are you ready?

Good, then read on.

You're thinking: "More food than I've ever eaten in my entire life! How?" It's no empty promise, but you'll have to read on to see it spelled out. For now, just trust me. It's a lot of eating, and it's all in the cause of a great body.

I won't blame you if you ask: how long? How much time do you have to invest in being eighteen again? I won't promise a given age. I don't have to. But honestly, if you give me three months of your life, and do the things I say, you will never look back. That's how long it takes to embed the discipline into your everyday life. In three months it will be normal. In three months you won't want to approach life any other way. How do I know? Because I live that lifestyle.

That brings us to qualifications. What are mine? I'm not a nutritionist or a gym rat. I'm an Oral and Maxillofacial Surgeon. I am also a personal trainer but I don't practice this as a trade. I have earned my certificate in personal training from John P. Parrillo's *Parrillo Certified Fitness Training* program. Once again, I am not a nutritionist or a dietitian. I am simply someone who has trained, observed, and learned.

In getting my certificate in personal training I learned a ton about sports nutrition. I'm also an amateur, competitive bodybuilder, and I'm very good at it. My credentials are my championships. I typically win shows in which I compete for the Masters over-40 groups. I usually compete in the Mid-Atlantic States. The individuals who have mentored me are Cliff Sheets, Ph.D., a clinical nutritionist, and master trainer John Parrillo. Later I'll give you all the information about their products and literature, so you can fill in the blanks. My goal is to share with you all that they have taught me, so you too can finally reach your physique and health goals.

Though I am not a nutritionist, I do have a lecture series which I conduct nationwide. The series title carries the same name as this book: *Turning Back the Hands of Time*. Most often I lecture to medical or dental colleagues. My audiences are often made up of medical nutritionists and dieticians, and don't we have a good time! These individuals grill me.

Some of them suggest that I'm trying to teach everyone to be a bodybuilder. Nothing could be further from the truth. I'm simply teaching a plan for fitness and diet where a person can lose as much fat as they wish. The discussion usually ends when I ask them if they are truly happy with how they look. I ask if a loss of five or ten pounds of fat, and a ripped, sculpted physique is something they desire. The discussion usually ends there. But even if you're not trying to look like a champion, do you want to feel like one? And most importantly: do you want to have the energy, vitality and stamina that go with a strong, healthy physique? Few people in my audiences can deny the desire for these benefits.

But just as I can talk to them, I can talk to you. I'm a hard working stiff just like you. I've mentioned training, observation, and learning, but how did I put it all together? How do I know what works? Experience, reflection, and invention. Experience? My wife, Margie and I live this lifestyle. Reflection? I learned from others, but found the core of it within myself. Invention? I've thought about it, and systematized it so that I could explain it in print.

Yes I'm also disciplined, and organized about my life— a bit anal some may say— but you don't have to be a Type A personality to do this. You can be laid back, or different in a thousand ways. You need only have some inner discipline, enough for a healthy work ethic. If you haven't got that, this is not the right book for you. The lifestyle that you are about to embark upon does take work.

So you say: I spent my hard-earned money on this book, and now the jerk tells me I need discipline. Yes, you do. You need forty minutes of training three-to-four days a week, and seven hours of sleep a night. That's it.

Now you want to know: How does this nut expect forty minutes of training and seven hours of sleep in my already packed, overloaded, and squeezed-in day? I can't address those particulars. I can only say three things: first, good health and fitness come with a price; second, most of you who've read this far can do it; third, it will be worth it.

Do you have an IRA, or own any funds or stocks? I do also. These are our investments. They are our retirement. They are our future. I have a financial advisor, Dave. At this point he's laughing because he knows I can barely tell the difference between a mutual fund and a stock. Dave can, and that's why I listen to him. He knows finances. Nutrition and fitness are the most important investments you make. Good health is an investment in your future. Without your health you have nothing. I do know something about that, probably as much as Dave knows about finances.

As a surgeon my patients span the years. I see kids and I see great grandparents. Some patients come to me when they're in their sixties or seventies, and with age comes illness. They've saved all their lives for retirement; now it's here, and they're sick. How did they treat their bodies throughout their lives? Most were very active as kids. Many played sports in high school and a few played in college as well. Then came jobs, kids, stress and the day-to-day ravages of poor nutrition and lack of exercise. Sugary breakfasts were followed by missed lunches, fatty snacks, and most days ended with a rich dinner. What's the outcome? Diabetes, coronary heart disease, hypertension, peripheral vascular disease, congestive heart disease, stroke, arthritis, etc… i.e serious debilitating illness—all from inattention. Why get sick from something you can avoid? Why save money for the future, only to let your health go to crap?

Forty minutes a day three to four days a week—it's non-negotiable. It's your daily investment for the future. It won't make you invulnerable. One day a massive aneurysm may take you on a 500-pound squat, but would you prefer Type II Diabetes to knock you off because you couldn't put down that last cream puff?

How long have you been looking at yourself in the mirror and wondering: "What has become of that sexy gal or guy that I used to be?" Are you sick of it? Are you tired of not being able to look at that reflection without asking: How on earth have I let this happen to me? What will it take to turn my life around? What will bring back my health? What will return me to the physique I should have? That's where I can help.

Just remember: it's a lifestyle change, not a pill; it's a commitment, not a miracle two-minute exercise machine off of a midnight infomercial. If those things worked America would be a nation of bodybuilders: huge ripped guys in shorts and tanks, and firm-toned gals with perfect butts in thongs. But look out the window! We're the most obese nation in the world. As a mentor once told me: the American food industry is trying to kill us all with processing, preservatives and fats.

Why aren't we a nation of healthy muscular maniacs? After all, it seems like almost every American diets, orders an Ab Cruncher, joins a cut-down-on-calories club or goes to the local gym. So why are we still fat? What's the secret?

Shhhh! Don't say it too loud, but the secret is: nutrition! Healthy Nutrition is the key to your exercise plan. How important is nutrition to your exercise plan? Is it 10%, 50%, or 60%? I would say it's 80%. Without healthy nutrition you will never achieve your goals. Without the right food you'll never see the peak; simple as that. But healthy nutrition doesn't mean less nutrition. Let's all say it together: I'm going to eat more food that I've ever eaten in my entire life!

I admit, I do this to the hilt: the competition level. This is not to say you should. It's only to say that I went into it with that as a barometer. When I began to compete I used to think: Why would anyone eat like this unless they're doing what I'm doing? That was before my first competition. After that the diet gradually became habit. Like any habit it snuck up on me. Before I knew it six months had passed, and I was still eating the best, most nutritious food that I could find. I never turned back. I don't miss how I used to eat. I hardly remember how I used to eat.

People often ask me how I maintain such a strong tight midsection, *i.e.* the six-pac abs. They think the rule on this is to do crunches at least once a day, but I don't. I work my abs out once every week or two. It's an exercise I hate! So how do I keep them so ripped? Everyone has rectus abdominis and lateral oblique musculature in their mid-sections. When there is no overlying fat, these muscles show. A ripped abdomen is simply a product of cardiovascular exercise and healthy diet, nothing more, nothing less. Buying that ab cruncher or doing a hundred sit-ups a day ain't gonna do it without the proper diet. Diet is the essential background to everything else.

That's why we're going to do first things first. Let's talk nutrition since it's my favorite subject and the foundation of all successful exercise plans.

Chapter II

THE PLAN THAT WILL FINALLY WORK!

T o pull a lot of my nutritional and philosophical ideas together, I'd like to begin Chapter II with a short aside: My wife, Margie and I recently went to my best friend, Bruce's house for dinner. Two weeks earlier I had won the overall championship for the Maryland State Cup Bodybuilding Competition. I was being particularly careful about what I ate because the Mr. Maryland Competition was only four weeks away. This was my cheat meal for the week, one where I give myself some leeway. Prior to dinner I was talking with Bruce's wife Yvette, a beautiful woman of Cuban heritage who is also an employee of mine. Yvette is a hell of a cook and homemaker. My own wife is also from a Caribbean culture: The Dominican Republic. These were our contexts as our conversation turned to diet.

About two years ago Bruce, a high-powered executive from Black and Decker, had had enough. He wanted to change his life. I got him started on my diet plan, increasing his calories (clean calories), cardiovascular, and strength-training exercise. He lost a ton of fat. Shortly after however he stopped and tried something new, *Body For Life* a diet-and-exercise plan sponsored by a nutritional supplement company. It was sweeping the country at that time. It was short lived, but he seemed to be doing alright. From there he went to the *South Beach Diet Plan*. From what I've learned, that one requires no exercise at all, but Bruce did have the good sense to keep up with his cardio and strength training exercises.

As Yvette and I talked, our conversation turned to Bruce's weight loss. I noted that, although he was much slimmer than he had been, his core (midsection) was still smooth and soft. I emphasized the nature of the weight he'd lost. This is as important as the weight itself. Was he losing fat? Lean mass (muscle)? Or water? On these other diets, Bruce had been losing more fluid and lean tissue than fat. He was keeping some of what he should've lost, and losing pounds he needed. If you lose the pounds you need, you're losing good health.

Our dinner consisted of imported Brazilian beef marinated in rock salt, Cuban beans and brown rice (one of my favorites), a Caesar salad— dressing mixed in— and a fruit salad for dessert. I chuckled when Yvette stated that this South Beach diet plan had become an entrenched life style. From her comment, and the meal, I could see why Bruce's mid-section was still a bit soft.

To understand why we should dissect the dinner:

Red meat once a week is a great idea: high quality protein dense nutrition. Cuban red beans and brown rice: legumes and complex carbohydrates are a combo that couldn't be better. But the Caesar salad, along with the dressing is a disaster.

We've taken perfectly beautiful fibrous carbohydrates and ruined them with a high fat dressing. A better option would have been to have the salad greens by themselves and the dressing on the side. Don't get me wrong, I love dressing but the way to eat it is to take a bite of the greens and simply touch the fork in the dressing to get the flavor.

They had fruit salad for dessert. You may hate me for this, but I didn't eat any. I remembered the upcoming Mr. Maryland competition, and stayed away. Melons, apples and bananas are not on our meal plan.

Finally we come to the beverages: beer for the men, pina coladas for the women. First it must be stated: no alcohol is good. To state it clearly, alcohol is an empty simple sugar with negative nutritional value. Beer and dark hard liquors like rums are the worst. During my cheat meal, I stick to straight vodka, distilled spirits from potatoes or grain, the cleanest alcohol there is. In fact, vodka and tequilla are the only distilled liquors with no carbohydrates. I'll also be willing to drink red wine fermented from grapes. Wine is not the best thing for you, but there is some cardiovascular benefit to a glass of red wine. Then there are those Pina Coladas. I won't say you can't have one, but understand this: mixing alcohol with fruit juices or sugary sodas is absolutely prohibited except during your cheat meal.

So how did this evening go? Let me preface this by saying that if my buddy, Bruce, had consistently followed my plan for the last two years, instead of bouncing from one fad to another, he would be rock solid by now.

After dinner we went downstairs to Bruce's basement gym. There I reminded him of certain exercises and his cardiovascular training plan. It seemed to get him back on track.

In the course of the evening, Yvette made an argument that to be successful my plan had to make the nutrition portion desirable to the masses. I agree, but I will qualify it with this remark: the self-disciplined masses. Only those who have tried other plans, and made their own efforts—and who have a degree of self-discipline—will want to do what it takes. Only when all else has failed, and the urge to make a long lasting change outweighs the momentary appetites, will this work. With *Turning Back the Hands of Time*, your diet will quickly become enjoyable. There's plenty of variety in the foods themselves, and a variety of ways to prepare them. And get this: you get to eat more food than you ever thought possible. With some work, willpower, and a little imagination, you will soon see that this is *the plan that will finally work.*

I see it so often: people who train and train with no results. I was one of them until five years ago. Why? Because I didn't know how to eat. This will sound crazy to anyone who sees any diet in terms of cutting down on foods, but my main problem was that I wasn't eating enough. Most people who follow an exercise plan, but don't get the results they want and need, aren't eating enough. Yep that's what I said: not eating enough. It's a simple proposition: with the right exercise, the more you eat the stronger you become. From this it follows that, as long as you're eating more of the right things, the more fat you loose, the leaner you become, and the younger you become. You may not be younger by the calendar, but you will feel younger, and most of you will look younger as well. Now you're saying: What is he talking about? How can I eat more and loose fat? The key word here is: fat.

Every other diet plan, whether it's a corporate program, a book you picked up at the drugstore, or some instructions from your overweight friend, is essentially dieting aimed at restricting calories. The idea is: less is better. That idea is wrong, and, as many of you know from experience, it leaves you as far from your goals as you were when you started.

Today most dieters are following some variation of a popular "low carb" or "no carb" diet. This is nuts. Carbohydrates are our energy sources. I tell someone this, and he argues back: "Dr. Emmett, I lost sixty pounds on this diet." It could be sixty or 160—it still doesn't answer the important questions:

- •What was your body composition prior to going on your "carb-free" diet?
- •What exactly did you loose? Fat, lean mass, or water?
- •How heart healthy was it? Could you eat a pound of bacon because it was "carb-free?" Your cardiovascular system will thank you all the way to the operating room.

Initially, this diet didn't even want its followers to eat fibrous carbohydrates *i.e.* vegetables. This ridiculous notion was eventually moderated and with good reason because it is invariably going to slow the peristaltic motion of your lower gastrointestinal track. That means that toxic waste products in your stool will hang around in your large intestine and colon setting the stage for colon cancer. Do you want to follow a diet plan that may contribute to cardiovascular and colon diseases? Thanks, but no thanks.

DR. JOHN EMMETT

The *South Beach Diet* book and all of the others aren't on my reading list. I look at and listen to people who follow them, and what I see are temporary, empty changes. I read nutrition journals, and follow the progress of scientific information and controlled experimentation.

❦ ❦ ❦

I finished writing this chapter over spring break, my one week off a year, during a vacation with my family. A Canadian man who we'd met earlier in the trip came up to our dinner table and commented on what a beautiful wife and handsome family I had. Countless times during the vacation, on the beach, and at the resort gym, people would comment on how great I looked and how they couldn't believe I was forty-two years old. These were complete strangers! They were envious of Margie and me. They admired our level of health and fitness. When was the last time you felt comfortable at the beach? When did you wear a bikini? Or take off your shirt? Has it been a while? I thought so! How would you like people to wish they were as lean and fit as you? Does that sound good? Well, your quest has just begun.

Sometimes I wonder if my kids aren't a little embarrassed about their mom and dad. Their parents look different from others. We don't fit into that obese unhealthy life. And what about kids? How do they fit into this mix of nutrition and fitness? I've spent countless hours listening to lecturers discuss nutrition. They all emphasize how important it is for kids to eat the same healthy foods as the parents. This is a fallacy. Don't get me wrong, children should learn the importance of a healthy diet, but face it: kids are kids and they need to eat like kids.

Children's metabolic rates are so much faster then ours that they can afford to have treats in addition to a well-balanced diet. As long as a child remains active with sports and play he or she can afford to eat just about anything. But remember: television and video games don't qualify as sports and play. Adolescent obesity is a serious problem in this country. The main cause of this is not poor diet habits, it's inactivity. It's too easy for kids these days to pass their time engaged in activities with little or no physical component.

High tech video games seduce children into sitting in one place, and performing mindless tasks. Although I have them in my home, I limit their use. The things I stress with my own children are education and sports. I personally coach two youth baseball teams and four youth soccer teams, (two outdoor and two indoor). In my opinion every child who is able, should be involved with sports, whether they like them or not. With the variety of physical activities available, your child is bound to enjoy and excel at something. If the first choice doesn't work, keep trying; sooner or later they will find one they like.

One temptation for parents is to allow recreation councils and sports programs to become babysitting services. Don't let that happen. You'll find that if you get involved your children will enjoy the sport more. You don't have to be a coach, just be there for the practices and the games. Volunteer to keep score, or bring snacks, or be a coach's helper. If a child is overweight and it is not due to a medical condition it's usually due to inactivity. Don't fall into this trap.

An obese child is far more likely to become an obese adult, with all the tragedy that causes. Many adult or adolescent systemic illnesses stem from childhood obesity. One tragic result is diabetes. The effects of this disease can be mitigated or eliminated entirely with more exercise. So again, keep them active.

Sports in general, and especially team sports build character, while impressing on a young mind that activity and health consciousness are good. This lasts a lifetime. And there's always that outside chance that the child you put on the baseball diamond at six years old will grow up to be an NCAA shortstop with a full college scholarship!

Feed your kids a healthy diet with quality proteins, complex starches, fibrous carbohydrates, fruits and dairy products. And those occasional hot dogs, chicken nuggets, pizza, ho-hos, twinkies, and ding dongs are okay.

All this talk about twinkies and ho-hos gets me hungry. Let's get back to the reason you bought this book: getting into the best shape of your life. What would you do to have sculpted muscle definition that turns heads, and an overall feeling of wellbeing beyond your wildest imagination? Would you pay ten thousand dollars? Would you change what you put in your body? Would you eat more? Would you alter your nutrition? Because, once again, that's the answer: nutrition, nutrition, nutrition.

Someone once said you are what you eat. Until about five years ago, I didn't believe it, but since then I've come to see that as the most brilliant statement ever made. If you eat crap you're going to look and feel like crap, both mentally and physically.

If you are in bad shape, and you eat the wrong combinations of food you will have to be ready for a radical change. If you can do that, read on. If not, this is as good a stopping point as any. Those of you who don't mind carrying around enough useless pounds to affect a healthy lifestyle simply aren't ready. Maybe you will never be. But don't throw the book away. Someday you may get tired of your present lifestyle. At that point you can pick it up again. It will still be valid.

As we begin to discuss nutrition, I'm going to tell you two things—the most important things. Some of you may know about one or both of these issues. Others may not. Trust me: they are critical in our quest.

First, we don't care about weight loss. Our goal is FAT LOSS. In fact most people who read this manual probably need to gain weight or stay at the same weight they are now. My goal is transformation: adding lean mass and losing fat. This is a question of body composition not measured by weight loss. It's measured by body stating. Body stating is a series of nine caliper measurements on various parts of the body plugged into a formula to determine your balance of body fat

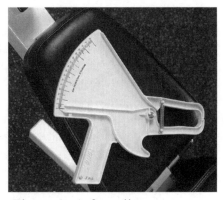

Figure 1- A fat caliper

vs. lean body mass (muscle).

Second, calorie-restrictive diets are counterproductive. When I tell you the more food you eat the more fat you lose, it sounds crazy but it's true. Why? Because of metabolism. Think of your body simply as a machine. The more fuel you give a machine the faster it runs; in the case of the body, the higher the metabolic rate will be. Conversely the less fuel you eat the slower your metabolism. With a low caloric intake your body recognizes a famine situation and shuts the motor down—exactly what we don't want to happen! We want to increase the nutrients to our bodies to feed the muscles which we are stressing during exercise so they can heal and hypertrophy (grow). At the same time this increase in our metabolic rate will help burn fat.

It may be true that the last time you dieted you lost weight. So what? What did you lose? Probably lean muscle and water. And because your body was in a starvation metabolic mode it hoarded as much fat as it could. What happened when you stopped that diet and resumed your normal dietary intake? Weight gain. Yep, it's called rebound fat gain. Forced into a slow metabolic rate your body hoarded even more fat. This process continued when the body was given more caloric opportunity.

Good nutrition and lots of quality calories is what we want. This will stimulate lean tissue growth and fat loss. On an average I'll consume 5-6 thousand calories over five meals. Normally I'll carry 6% - 7% body fat. Pre-competition I'll bump the calories to seven thousand for a few weeks, and really dial down to 4.8%-5 % body fat. In essence, I increase my calories to lose that last bit of subcutaneous fat (fat under the skin).

Calorie restrictive diets are counterproductive to what we are trying to achieve—physique perfection and long term health.

Chapter III

THE BODY BASICS

Over the years that I've been training and eating appropriately I've been questioned about what and how to eat. I truly feel that people want to eat healthy and correctly, but they simply don't know how. My goal is to teach you the correct way to eat for health, while avoiding the garbage.

As I drove to work one recent morning I heard a syndicated radio show where a panel was talking about overeating and obesity. They weren't advocating obesity, but every member of the panel was then, or had at one time been obese. They reported that the two biggest joys in life were eating and sex. I agree wholeheartedly with both. Believe you me, if you and your spouse or significant other eat clean and turn your bodies into beautiful healthy physiques, increased sexual enjoyment will follow.

With that in mind, let's look at the other part of the equation: eating. Eating can also be one of life's most joyous activities, but to enjoy it to the hilt you must be healthy. Almost everyone has noticed loss of appetite at the onset of a cold, flu, or other sickness. At these times even the scent of food makes some people nauseous. When you're merely out of shape you might think you're loving every bite you eat, but that just means that if you were truly healthy you'd love it even more. You'll find plenty of great tasting food on this journey, but remember, great taste is what lures us to the primary purpose of eating: nutrition.

What is nutrition? Nutrition is the food we put in our bodies, *i.e.* the nutrients. These are broken down into the following categories: Proteins, Carbohydrates, Fats, Vitamins, Minerals, and Water (a separate category).

Protein is a macronutrient. It's found in virtually all tissues of the body. It is essential in promoting growth and repair of tissues. Study after study also reports that protein intake can boost the metabolic rate by as much as 30%. However, the type of protein we choose to consume is critical. Proteins are made up of compounds called amino acids. There are twenty amino acids. Twelve of these are nonessential because our bodies produce them. Eight amino acids are essential, *i.e.* we need to get them from the foods we eat. I won't list all the amino acids but there are a few we need to know about: Leucine, Isoleucine, and Valine. These are Branched Chain Amino Acids (BCAAs), and they are the key to our success. BCAAs stimulate protein synthesis and are metabolized to produce lean muscular energy. All three BCAAs are essential and are readily available in the proteins found in our food. Our goal is to consume between 1.0 and 1.5 grams of protein per pound of body weight per day. This should be separated over five to six meals.

Which types of protein will we choose to eat? I bet you can guess. Yep, lean protein and plenty of it, high in clean calories and amino acids (especially BCAAs). I recommend white chicken or turkey breast, fish (including tuna), egg whites (the best source of lean protein i.e. pure albumin), shellfish, and red meat (probably the densest source of protein). Let's clarify something. Your white protein sources are your best. I eat red meat but reserve it to one meal per week, (usually my cheat meal). Although the density of protein in red meat is high, as is its iron concentration, the amino acid sequence and the high fatty content profile of red meat is very similar to that of humans. That makes it much easier for the body to compartmentalize red meat fat into human fat: the process of Nutrient Partitioning.

The process of Nutrient Partitioning is best explained by an example. Compare a root beer float made of vanilla ice cream and sugary soda to a chicken breast, broccoli salad and half a sweet potato. Each contains 700 calories but the body processes each meal differently. The ice cream soda is full of processed simple sugars which are quickly compartmentalized into fat. The natural protein, fibrous carbohydrate and starchy carbohydrate of the chicken, broccoli and sweet potato have a hard time being compartmentalized or partitioned into anything but lean mass and waste. You don't have to be a rocket scientist to figure out which one is better for you.

Proteins have a direct relationship to the metabolism. Besides building and repairing tissues, they also produce antibodies for the immune system, and enzymes and catalysts essential for nearly all metabolic reactions. Protein sources can be used for energy but that's exactly what we don't want to happen. Our protein supply should be used for building lean tissue. We want it for building, not burning.

Normally the body strikes a good balance between protein breakdown and protein synthesis, i.e. nitrogen balance. That balance should shift to synthesis (*anabolism,* or protein building) during growth periods like childhood, pregnancy, or healing. A negative protein (nitrogen) balance, (*catabolism*, or protein breakdown) occurs during injury or illness. It's also a prime feature of my favorite subject: caloric or carbohydrate restrictive diets.

Tell me how we can build lean muscle tissue and lose fat when our metabolic rate is down, our carbohydrates are restricted, and we're breaking down whatever proteins we're taking in for energy? For gosh sakes, carbohydrates are our best energy sources. Not protein! We can't gain lean muscle if we're using all our proteins as a less efficient energy source. Caloric-and-carb-restrictive diets are counter productive. Our goal is to gain muscle.

Remember muscle tissue is the most metabolically active tissue in the body. The more you produce the more activity goes on in your body. Simply increasing your lean muscle mass increases the metabolic rate of that mass, thus burning body fat! On a caloric-and-carb restrictive diet you lose weight by losing lean tissue and water. Your metabolic rate drops, your body hoards fat, and you lose muscle tissue. Again, not rocket science. Let's move on to carbohydrates our second macronutrient.

When I was a kid, I was a big Clint Eastwood fan. His breakthrough movie was *The Good, the Bad, and the Ugly*. That title describes carbohydrates as well. There are good complex carbohydrates, which we need as sources of energy. There are bad carbohydrates which we should avoid at all cost. Then there are the ugly carbohydrates which we should be ashamed to even put in our mouths.

Glucose is the final product of all carbohydrate metabolism. Glucose is also our primary source of energy. What we don't use, we store in the liver and muscle tissue as glycogen: stored energy or we convert it to fat.

Let's call our bad and ugly carbohydrates sugars. What are sugars? They can be building blocks for our good carbohydrates: polysaccharides or complex carbohydrates. Or they can be agents of catastrophe. The difference lies in how these are digested and metabolized.

When I began my amateur bodybuilding career, I competed against a young man whom we'll call Bill. Bill owned a gym and was a personal trainer. In my first competition he beat me badly. After that, all I wanted to do for my next competition was emulate Bill.

In the meantime, I met John Parrillo, who has a fitness training program. John recommended that I read his training and nutrition manual. He also suggested that I read *Lean Bodies* by Dr. Cliff Sheets. I read them both. The next year I entered the same competition hard as a rock, with paper thin skin. Again, I was competing against Bill. I beat him, and won the competition for the Over-35 Masters Division. Both of these books are available by calling 1-800-344-3404.

My discussion with Bill that day led to carbohydrate metabolism and digestion. Bill's belief was that because all carbohydrates were metabolized into glucose, a carbohydrate was a carbohydrate was a carbohydrate. Boy, was he wrong. So are others who advocate "low-carb" or "no-carb" diet plans.

Sugars are simple carbohydrates. There are a number of different sugars, but all are digested and metabolized in the same fashion. There are two classes of sugars: monosaccharides and disaccharides.

Monosaccharides are the simplest forms of sugar. They include glucose which we've discussed, fructose which is found in fruit as "fruit sugar," and galactose found in milk.

Disaccharides are two monosaccharides linked together. Sucrose, which is table sugar, is glucose and fructose linked together. It is commonly found in sugar cane, maple sugar and pineapple. Maltose is malt sugar found in cereal grains. It is glucose and glucose linked together. Lactose is milk sugar. It is glucose and galactose linked together. It is the only natural sugar found in animal products. The use of milk throughout life is a strangely human practice. No other mammal chooses to drink milk after weaning. This may be one reason that we don't see many obese deer or pudgy mountain lions. Why do we choose milk over water?

A discussion of the digestion and metabolism of sugars exposes them as "the bad and the ugly" carbohydrates. These carbs pass through the digestive system virtually untouched, coming to rest in the small intestine. They are broken down by the gastrointestinal system and also pass into the small intestine. Becoming single molecules, the monosaccharides are absorbed rapidly into hepatic portal system and pass to the liver. With this rapid absorption of sugar, *i.e.* glucose, into the blood stream the pancreas is stimulated to quickly release a hormone called insulin. Insulin's main function is to drive glucose molecules into the cells of the body tissues to be used for energy. The liver converts monosaccharides such as fructose and galactose into glucose. Excess glucose is stored in the liver and skeletal muscle as glycogen, long chains of glucose molecules that can be used later for energy.

But let's consider what happens if no excessive energy is burned, *i.e.* no cardiovascular or strength-training exercise is being performed. How much glucose will be stored as glycogen? Very little. So with the rapid absorption of these carbs, and the sharp spike of insulin release, where does the excess glucose go? It is rapidly converted to fat and stored in the fat cells of the body.

And let me tell you, once it's in the fat cells it's extraordinarily difficult to get out.

To continue with our Clint Eastwood analogy, what about the "good" carbohydrates? These are complex carbohydrates or polysaccharides. Poly means "many," so a polysaccharide is multiple monosaccharides linked together into a long, chain-like complex molecule. These complex polysaccharides make up our starchy carbohydrates.

Some starchy carbohydrates are potatoes, rice (especially brown rice), sweet potatoes, oatmeal, lima beans, yams, corn and legumes. These complex polysaccharides are also all broken down into glucose. But if that's true, you ask, how can they be any different from simple sugars? It's all a function of digestion and metabolism.

What's the difference between simple sugar and complex polysaccaharide metabolism? It's the rate at which the body processes them. Simple sugars are digested, absorbed, and the excess are stored in the fat cells in the wink of an eye. Complex carbohydrates take their time. Because they are extremely long chains it takes awhile for them to work their way through the gastrointestinal tract, then to be absorbed into the bloodstream. This digestive process requires more energy because it is slow. Insulin is released slowly as well. This gradual release of insulin assures that most glucose goes only to the tissues which need energy the most.

Later you'll see how the skeletal muscles receive the majority of this energy-producing glucose, where it is used or stored as glycogen. The liver will also store glycogen.

To recap:

The right kind of carbs are "the Good"—no matter what the others say. The right kind are starchy complex carbohydrates: the polysaccharides. These turn up in your kitchen as brown rice, oatmeal, potatoes, yams, legumes, lima beans, corn and many other good foods.

The wrong kind, "the Bad and the Ugly," are processed sugary carbohydrates i.e. monosaccharides and disaccharides—the most difficult kind to avoid. They roll through our supermarkets and restaurants like camouflaged tanks, running roughshod over the best of our intentions. You have to be very careful. For gosh sakes, read labels! It's the best way to dodge them. If the label indicates high sugar content put the item back on the shelf.

One note: I told you I don't read fad diet books, but Margie occasionally looks at them. She borrowed one of the most recent popular trendy diet books from a friend. While I was writing this I flipped the book open and looked up potatoes. Their exact words on the subject were: "They have to go." So now I reiterate: "They have to stay!" They're too good a source of energy to pass up. With our exercise program, and the rest of our diet, you'll need these potatoes as an energy source. The current fad diets will pass like all the others before them, but potatoes are forever.

There's even a plan based upon the Lord. They ask you to pray in the morning, eat as if it were biblical times, and rub cleansing oils into your hands. In forty days you're a new person.

I'm sure it's a good plan, and if you want to be the person they describe fine. If you want something more down-to-earth you have to work for it. So, for those that can, follow my regimen. Exercise hard and eat clean. I doubt that the Lord will object to that.

Now, let me answer a few fallacies:

Are any of you saying: "High carbs? That's heresy!" Let me give you another one: Where do we find a ton of sugar? (You'll hate this!) In fruit and dairy products. Sorry. Fruit and dairy products are full of fructose and galactose. I went four years without eating fruit, but six months ago I felt I was running my glycemic index a bit low. I began with a handful of berries in the morning with breakfast. I choose berries because they have a high content of antioxidants. I focus mostly on blueberries and raspberries. I've found that they haven't hurt me a bit. They may even provide me a bit more fullness to my physique as I go into competition. (Or is that my imagination?) So I'm not completely discounting all fruits and dairy products. Fruits and dairy products are full of minerals, and vitamins which are excellent for your health, but— and this is a big "but"—they're full of simple sugar which is rapidly compartmentalized as fat.

I limit my dairy products to a splash of fat free milk in my coffee in the A.M. and a piece of fat free cheese once every other day or so. That's it. Coffee, you say? What's he doing taking caffeine? A vice or two in moderation anchors any diet. I'm human, you know.

Tons of fruit, yogurt and fat free milk are not the way to the healthy physique of your dreams.

I know you ladies are thinking—Where am I going to get my calcium for strong bones and teeth if I eliminate dairy products. I'll tell you. Fish, legumes (of all types), and leafy green vegetables. Ladies, there's as much calcium in a good healthy salad as there is in a glass of milk!

❦ ❦ ❦

I have a buddy named Ron. He's a forty-something father whose kids go to school with mine. Gail, his wife of twenty years is something special, and if you saw her you'd know instantly why Ron is so interested in getting in the best shape possible.

Ron came to my house, and while he was there he started looking over my gym and my competitive trophies. The sight of all that got him pumped up. I had just explained to him that cardio exercise done first thing in the morning was the best method for fat loss. Ron looked, listened, and was psyched.

He said, "John, from now on I'm going to wake up, drink a big glass of juice, and go out for a run."

"Hold it right there," I said. I took him to the fridge and pulled out the carton of OJ we keep for our kids, then I walked over to the pantry and got a pack of Reese's Cups.

"Take a look," I said, pointing out the sugar content listed on each label.

Ron read the labels and blinked. "There's more sugar in a cup of OJ then there is in the Reese's cups."

That was Ron's education. Go to your kitchen, and you'll probably find similar educational material. When you do, don't let anyone tell you that the sugar in juice is healthier then the sugar in a Reese's Cup or any candy for that matter. I see it like this: sugar in candy is a disaccharide and fructose is a monosaccharide, so fruit sugar will be absorbed faster than candy sugar creating a faster insulin spike, and a faster deposit into fat. So is candy sugar better then fruit sugar? Probably not, but there's no need to include either one in our diet for ultimate physique.

Now that we've scored a knockout on the sugar and complex carbohydrates, let's go for the real deal: breads and pastas. Though these are not quite "ugly" I will fit them into the "bad" category. Why? Today's breads and pastas lack nutritional value.

Though you've probably heard this before, I want to put it as bluntly as I can: The US food industry processes and preserves all the flour products available to us. None of the flour or bread products available to us today have any nutritional value. The nutritious value in the grain coverings have been manipulated and preserved. But, you think, I only buy whole grain enriched bread products with no preservatives. Look at that thought. The only positive thing in it is that there are no preservatives. An enriched grain is a processed grain, and as for the wholeness of it: where is its covering? But isn't it enriched with vitamins and minerals? Yes, after they have processed out all the natural vitamins and minerals. Once the US food industry is done with them bread and pasta products are no more than rapidly absorbable simple carbohydrates. That's food for fat.

I seldom eat either. I may have a bite of a dinner roll during my weekly cheat meal but that's it. I don't eat sandwiches nor do I eat plates full of pasta.

By now you're wondering what planet I'm from. I assure you I'm from right here on Earth. If you are what you eat, I'm from what I believe is the best the Earth has to offer. Give it a little time and I think you'll agree. Read on, follow the program, and in six weeks when you look in a mirror you'll see what I mean. Already your body will have undergone a metamorphosis. When you've got six weeks of habit-building discipline under your belt, and you see how that belt fits on your new body, you won't miss the triple-decker sandwich—at least not enough to trade that body for it. Then you are closing in on an entirely new life style.

Are you still looking up at the sky, trying to catch a glimpse of my spaceship? Ok, I'll make a deal with the ones who don't think they'll be able to stand the change: add a minimal bit of fruit and breads. But this deal doesn't come without strings: "minimal" means just that. The intake of these products should be limited to a small handful of berries a day and bread or pasta no more then once or twice a week, *i.e.* one or two meals. Remember we're eating 35 meals per week. Make sure the fruits are low glycemic, and for gosh sakes nothing but whole grain breads and pastas.

You might start believing that I'm from right here on our native Earth when I bring up the other good carbohydrates. These are the fibrous carbohydrates, in other words: vegetables. From my point of view any vegetable is a healthy vegetable. Roots, greens, stalks, spears—they all have their place in the diet. I have favorites. Sometimes I think I'm going to turn into a stalk of asparagus. No matter, I know it's good for me.

Fibrous carbohydrates provide some calories and energy, but this is not their main function. Fiber assists intestinal function and elimination of waste. It provides bulk to our diets. Examples of fibrous carbohydrates are skins of fruits, vegetables, and the coverings of cereal grains. Other fibrous carbohydrates include broccoli, green peas, beans, lettuce, peppers, and asparagus. Again, all vegetables are good. Eat as many of them as possible. If it's green eat it! The normal American diet lacks fiber, and this leads to gastrointestinal abnormalities, such as constipation, diverticulitis, irritable bowel syndrome, and colon cancer.

I've got to tell you a story. Yesterday I took my son to the Orioles game. We had seats behind a thirty-something couple. I don't say this to be cruel, but only to be accurate. The husband was overweight and his wife was morbidly obese. My son and I left in the bottom of the seventh inning, but what we had witnessed before that was an all too common process.

The young lady ordered a plateful of cheese nachos and a regular coke. That's enough extras for me for a year, but she was just getting started. The next inning, it was a Philly Cheese steak, with two packets of mayo. She devoured that in less then an inning. I had a hard time ignoring this food fest, but I managed to get back into the 4-4 tie on the field.

In the fifth, it was a bag of cotton candy which she had stashed away in her bag. During the sixth inning, the woman summoned the waitress again, wanting a bag of peanuts and another coke. In less than two hours this woman had consumed enough fat and sugar to start a candy factory.

There I was worrying about all the sodium and white rice I'd taken in with the six pieces of sushi I'd eaten and the quarter-bag of sunflower seeds my son and I had shared before the game. I guess guilty pleasures are a relative thing.

I tell you about this young lady for a reason. She is not alone. Her ballgame food binge is the norm in America. To put it bluntly, we are a nation of fat slobs, but we keep that knowledge at arm's length. Do you think this obese woman knows why she's obese? Does she understand the central fact that's visible to anyone who sees her? I doubt it. Will she understand what she's inflicted on herself and her familywhen she's diagnosed with heart disease, hypertension, and/or diabetes within just a few short years? Only she can say.

But if we are to become anything but a nation of bloat we have to change that behavior. Lose the cheese steak subs and cotton candy, and soon I'll want you to advance to feeling a twinge of guilt about white rice, (even if it isn't the worst alternative for a complex carb), and salted sunflower seeds. That kind of attitude may seem light years away, but you can get there in a few weeks. Trust me, follow me, and it will happen. Once you see and feel your transformation there's no looking back.

Our next topic is fats. As with carbohydrates, these aren't a one-size-fits-all. We have good fats and bad fats. We'll figure out what the good fats are, then limit ourselves to a fat consumption of 5-to-10 %.

If you skim the surface of the media—headlines, spam headings in email, and the loudest voices on TV and radio—you get the feeling that any diet should start with low fats. Ever since nutrition became a popular science we've been fed the idea that fat is bad. That's not always the case.

Fats are present in one form or another in most foods. Fats are also vital to life. Foods like red meats and dairy products are highest in fats.

Fats have numerous functions. Fat soluble vitamins are transported by fats, and are essential for life. Fats are a source of energy. Fats insulate the body, protect our organs, aid in temperature regulation, and healthy nerve function.

Two of the most important fats are Linolenic (Omega -3) and Linoleic (Omega-6), the Essential Fatty Acids (EFAs). The body does not produce these so we must get them from our diets. Found most often in the fats and oils of vegetables and fish, they are critical. The EFAs should make up 2% of our body's caloric intake.

Lipids are another fat-like molecule in our bodies. There are three lipids, triglycerides, phospholipids and sterols. Triglycerides are the most common. Triglycerides are stored as fats when excessive calories are consumed. All triglycerides are similar in structure. They have three fatty acids linked by a glycerol molecule. Glycerol, a carbohydrate, can, when metabolized, be converted to glucose. The metabolizing of fatty acids depends on their chain length (short, medium or long) and their degree of saturation. Saturation of the fatty acids depends upon how many hydrogen atoms they carry. Mono and polyunsaturated fats have organic double bonds to satisfy their bonding requirements. The more a fatty acid is saturated the harder it is to metabolize and easier it is to be stored. Try your best to read labels and avoid saturated fatty acids.

Phospholipids are another abundant lipid which is vital for life. Phospholipids make up a large portion of the membranes of animals cells. Phospholipids have two fatty acid chains compared to triglycerides. The most common phospholipid in our bodies is lecithin, found in beans and eggs.

Sterols are the most notorious of the lipids. These include cholesterol, phytosterol (plant sterols) and steroid hormones. The most famous, cholesterol, comes from what we eat, and is manufactured by our bodies. It's found in virtually all of our tissues. Excessive cholesterol levels are usually associated with cardiovascular disease. The oxidation of cholesterol during metabolism makes it dangerous. Cholesterol levels are determined most by genetic predisposition and dietary fat intake, but even if you're predisposed to elevated cholesterol, as I am, you can keep it low by maintaining a low fat diet, concentrating on polyunsaturated fats. On our diet we discourage the intake of high cholesterol foods.

It's also important to identify LDL or (Low Density Lipoprotein) as bad cholesterol and HDL (High Density Lipoprotein) as good cholesterol. Lipoproteins enable lipids to circulate through the body. Lipids are insoluble in water and most are surrounded by proteins to be transported in the blood. Types of lipoproteins are identified by their densities: VLDLs are very low density lipoproteins, LDLs are low density lipoproteins, while HDLs are high density lipoproteins. VLDLs are manufactured in the intestine and liver. Their main function is to transport triglycerides and a small amount of cholesterol and phospholipids. As they transport the triglycerides to the tissues they become more like LDL. Most LDLs are formed in the liver. They carry cholesterol and some triglycerides, and phospholipids. They are considered bad because of their levels of cholesterol (50%). They create plaque on artery walls. The HDLs are the good lipoproteins which mostly transport phospholipids.

In a nutshell we've covered macronutrients.

Now we'll talk briefly about micronutrients: vitamins, minerals and water.

Vitamins are divided into two groups: water soluble vitamins and fat soluble vitamins. Vitamins don't provide energy but act as coenzymes which help convert macronutrients into metabolically active forms of energy. Coenzymes speed up the body's chemical reactions. Most vitamins are essential: they can't be manufactured by our bodies and must be obtained by our food or from supplements. No discussion of vitamins is complete without a mention of the American food industry, which has drained these essential micronutrients from most foods. What are these micronutrients?

The Essential Vitamins Are as Follows:
Fat Soluble: Vitamin A, D, E, and K.

Water Soluble: Niacin B3, Pantothenic Acid, Vitamin C (ascorbic acid), Vitamin B1 Thiamin, Vitamin B2 Riboflavin, Vitamin B6 Pyridoxime, Vitamin B12 Cobalamin, Biotin and Folic Acid.

The Fat Soluble vitamins are stored by the body. These vitamins are found in both plants and animal sources. They are measured in IU's or International Units.

The water soluble vitamins are not stored by the body. These must be regularly supplied by our nutrition. They are mostly found in vegetables. They are measured in milligrams or micrograms. Overcooking veggies can destroy a lot of these, so raw vegetables are your best bet for the water soluble vitamins.

ANTIOXIDANTS are free radical scavengers. Free radicals occur when cells become chemically unstable because of radiation, pollution, or normal body metabolism. Free radicals contain an extra electrical charge. They seek out neutralization. Once one is neutralized, another free radical is formed. This process goes on damaging cells until other substances neutralize the chain reaction. Free radical damage has been linked to processes of aging and cancer. Vitamins A, C, E, selenium, and superoxide dismutase are all antioxidants. Foods very high in antioxidants are berry fruits. One fruit I advocate in small portions is blueberries. It is probably the best fruit of all.

How do you know if you're getting enough vitamins? The best way is to take a multivitamin supplement. Looking at the RDA of all the processed foods on the market may not help you. Processing leaves most foods so low in vitamins and minerals that you may be kidding yourself.

If you're drinking plenty of water and your urine still has a light yellow tone you're probably getting enough vitamins and minerals. But remember, you have got to be well hydrated. In a dehydrated state your body won't make as much urine and it will be dark yellow. This is not a sign of adequate vitamin intake but simply of dehydration.

MINERALS are inorganic substances in their simplest forms: elements from the earth. Our bodies do not create minerals, but we need them. Minerals help complete the majority of organic chemical reactions in our bodies. These are essential for normal metabolic function. Minerals help maintain fluid balance in our bodies. They help with cognitive function, nerve transmission, muscle function etc.

Dr. John Emmett

The Essential Minerals Are as Follows:

Calcium, chloride, sodium, sulfur, potassium, magnesium, and phosphorus. These are macrominerals—we need a lot of these. Also essential are trace minerals, Iodine, Fluroide, Maganganese, Molybdenum, Nickel, Iron, Copper, Selenium, Silicon, Chromium, Cobalt, Vanadium, and Zinc. Though we don't need these in as high a quantity, they are necessary.

A side note on labels: All that sugar-free ice cream you've been eating isn't sugar-free. Corporations are not required to label sugar alcohols, *i.e.* glycerols, as sugars. Sugar alcohols are metabolized to glucose simply and rapidly. Don't be taken in by this "bait and switch" tactic. Be a label expert and scrutinize every product that you consider buying.

Water

Next to oxygen, water is the most important substance to life. It is involved in every bodily function. It makes up 60% of our body composition. It is the basis of our blood, sweat and tears, and is essential for nerve transmission, muscle function, circulation, digestion, respiration, and every heartbeat. We lose two quarts of water per day simply thru respiration, urine, and feces. Half of this is replaced by the foods we eat and half should be replaced by drinking water. Remember however, this is simply basal metabolism. If your job requires any activity at all, or if you live in a temperate climate your requirement will go up. Why? Because you will lose more water in the form of sweat. Adults should drink at least two quarts of water per day, and more is probably better.

A story about water might help you understand. Being an oral surgeon I treat a lot of serious facial infections stemming from bad teeth. These infections can be life-threatening. In addition to our modern antibiotics, one of my mainstays in treating these is a high-protein diet and plenty of water. When you are sick your doc always tells you to drink plenty of fluids. That's because you need to hydrate your body to allow it to fight the infection to the best of its ability. More importantly you dilute the infection out of your body, washing the bacterial cells or viral particles out of your system in the urine. And why am I recommending a high

Water plays an essential role in my training schedule before competitions. Ten days before competition I begin to drink heavily. I'm not talking about beer; I begin to drink water. In a ten-to-eleven hour work day I'll drink approximately three-to-four gallons of water per day. This hydrates me, and it also causes me to go into diuresis, or to urinate to excessive levels.

I urinate between patient visits throughout the day. Why is this important? It gets out every bit of the body fluid trapped under my skin. This is the pre-competition mode. Twelve hours prior to competition I stop drinking with the exception of sips of H^2O just to wet my whistle. That way my body is still in diuresis but I'm taking in no fluids. When I go up on stage I'm completely dehydrated and my skin is as thin as possible. Now is this what I advocate? Hell no! Don't even think about it. With all the super-hydration I also have to take electrolytes (i.e. the minerals we just spoke about). Hyponatremia (low sodium) or hypokalemia (low potassium) can be life threatening and are both associated with excessive fluid intake. This regimen is complex, and if you don't know what you're doing you can damage your body. I've seen people collapse on stage and be carried to hospitals for dehydration and electrolyte imbalance. But the process does make me acutely aware of the role water plays in the body. Nothing is more vital to health.

protein diet? To allow your body to produce antibodies to fight the infection.

I once had a patient who was on the verge of being admitted to the hospital so she could get IV antibiotics; she just wouldn't get better on oral antibiotics. I keep banging my head against the wall. I didn't get it. Again we went through all my instructions. I found out that she had substituted ice tea hydration rather than good old water. What did that do? The caffeine in the ice tea was a diuretic so she was becoming more dehydrated instead of less. Once we commenced with real superhydration (using water) she turned the corner within twenty-four hours. She didn't need to go to the hospital.

Never underestimate the power of water. This is one of the most important things I'll ever teach you. Drink, drink, drink, your water. But what do we Americans do? We drink fruit juices (sugar fluid), soda, (sugar and caffeine), ice tea (more caffeine), coffee (more caffeine), anything but water. Why? I have no idea. Maybe good old water is too plain. Don't let that stop you. Drink at least a half a gallon of water a day. It will make a huge difference!

Chapter IV

PUTTING IT ALL TOGETHER

This is the chapter where you learn how to eat, so here I repeat: Put down that fad diet book! I see them in supermarkets, drug stores, and bookstores, lined up like soldiers ready to storm your kitchen. They're huge, stretching like Russian novels across all those pages. How do they take up so much room? I'll tell you how—with a thousand five-minute meals, ten-day diets, resulting in twenty lost pounds. Then you gain it all back by the end of the month, and go buy the next diet book. It's a hell of a way to operate the human body.

In the last two chapters, I've told you about nutrition. In those brief pages are all the basics you need to know. With that solid background we can now learn how to eat.

In the question periods after my lectures, I'm often asked: "Dr. Emmett, what do you eat every day?" I always have fun answering. That's when the jaws start dropping. As I detail the meals and the food, they start shaking their heads. Usually somebody comes up with some variation of: "For God's sake, I could never do that."

It's not that they can't imagine eating the food, it's just that there are so many sweets, junk foods, fast foods, and empty foods that they eat every day. Those are nowhere to be found. And there's also so much. I'm talking about meal after meal after meal after meal, a whole lot of food, and it's not bird seed either. Chicken, tuna, potatoes, rice... even a great big steak now and then. And I haven't totally eliminated cheese, peanut butter or dressing on a salad. I've just cut most of the fat and sugar out of these.

There's so much! That's what you must remember when you want to stop defeatism in its tracks. Just find your positive imagination, and start applying it to your own life, your own kitchen, and your own body. If you can't get past "I can't" then why have you read this far? If you're feeling some residual doubts now, and that "I can't" voice is echoing in the back of your head, my response is: "Don't you want to eat more food than you have ever eaten in your entire life?"

It's not as hard as it sounds.

It's fun!

And as one of my buddies used to say, "You eat like a Roman!"

Put defeatism aside. Find the discipline inside yourself. You'll need a lot of it at first, but then you won't need as much, and finally it won't seem like "discipline" at all. Anyone can eat this way. There are a lot of different ways to do it. And if you truly want to change your life for the better, it will soon be easy. It just takes some getting used to.

On the other hand, if you are satisfied with looking in the mirror and seeing that gut hanging over your belt or your hips and butt looking like the bottom half of a pear, you obviously don't need to eat any differently than you do now. I think you get my point.

But let's go back to that question at my lecture: What do I eat every day? Today, after my two-mile run at 5:00 a.m., I ate a fifteen-egg-white omelet with vegetables, a bowl of oatmeal with blueberries and raspberries, a bowl of protein pudding and a protein shake. Seems like a lot? Hold on. At 9:30 a.m. I had a turkey salad, half a sweet potato, a bowl of protein pudding, a protein shake, and an energy bar. At 1:30 p.m. I ate tuna salad, half a sweet potato, protein pudding, another protein shake, and another energy bar. At 5:30 p.m., again, turkey salad, I skipped the potato and the energy bar here, though you wouldn't have to (I'm gearing up for a competition). To this I added protein pudding, and a protein shake. I came home and trained with weights for about twenty minutes. At about 9:30 p.m., I ate a barbecue chicken breast, a salad with no-fat dressing, steamed asparagus with broccoli and cauliflower.

Now you're saying: "My God, that is a lot of calories." Yes, but from eating all these calories and doing these little bits of cardiovascular and strength training exercise my metabolic rate is so high that I burn it right up. And look what I ate. There is not a simple sugar or low-quality fat in the bunch. It's all protein, complex carbohydrates, fibrous carbohydrates, and omega fatty acids. Exactly what your body needs to burn fat and become lean.

And these aren't the exact foods you have to eat. They're the ones I wanted today. They came from a wide variety of options, enough to fill a sizeable restaurant menu. Soon there will probably be restaurants with such menus, and they'll serve the healthiest, tastiest meals in town.

Shortly I'll show you how I prepared these meals, and the other ones I eat all week long. It'll be my way, which to me is exciting and different, but I'm sure all of you will find variations that will get that new restaurant going overnight. After all, no matter what the diet is, if it doesn't please the palate who's going to eat it? I wouldn't, and neither would you.

I'm not trying to address just bodybuilders or competitive athletes, and I can't tell you to change your diet overnight. Few can do that. So take your time. Just as there are various foods, there are also various methods to get into this. In the past I've used a couple of strategies when coaching folks who simply want to get into excellent shape.

These strategies that I use are called "Periodization." They have been used for years by athletes to slowly shape and change their nutritional intake.

Although there are many Periodization techniques, the two that I believe work the best are outlined below. These both allow a gradual approach to the Hands Of Time nutritional balance. By month two or three, when you've mastered these techniques, you've positioned yourself to make unbelievable progress.

Family, friends, and coworkers will be astounded by the changes in you. This positive reinforcement makes it even easier to clean up the diet even farther. Use it to scale down that next cheat weekend into a cheat meal, or to stretch that twenty-minute cardio session to thirty minutes, sprinting that last eighth of a mile, or to finally feel the challenge of the weights, blasting out those extra reps. That's when the plan becomes effortless; the cause-and-effect nature of the nutrition and exercise have become habitually fun.

For the first time in ages you feel alive. Your vibrancy, stamina, and endurance have exponentially increased.

We also haven't forgotten about taste. Your diet is so clean now that we can introduce sweet tasting high nutritional supplements. You don't need that candy bar, cup of yogurt or bag of chips. Now with each meal you're satisfying your sweet tooth with a high protein pudding, thick shake, or great tasting nutritional bar.

Sound like a dream? It isn't. Read on about Periodization, and choose the method to change your life forever.

Always keep in mind the four main food groups that we're trying to eliminate from our diets:

- sweet, sugary desserts and fruits
- dairy products
- bread and pasta
- fatty junky carbohydrates

PERIODIZATION I.

In the first month, pick one of these food groups each week, and eliminate only that one from your diet plan for that one week. You might start with the one you eat least of, and work up. (Of course, I won't let you start with one that you don't eat at all, so if you happen to be allergic to dairy products, replace these weeks with ten-day periods, or something comparable.) In the second month eliminate each food group for two weeks (thus always having two groups absent from the diet), then three groups per week in the third month, and by the fourth month you will be fully into the program. This is the easy way to go about it, but don't expect the changes to come as rapidly this way. Using this method the plan will work very slowly, but if you stick with it, it will do the job. By that fourth month, you'll be well on your way to a lean, fit body, especially with the cardiovascular and resistance exercises.

You know yourself, and your will power. If you feel you want to jump right in, but want a gradual approach try this:

PERIODIZATION II.

Eliminate all four food groups from your new diet plan Monday through Friday. On Saturday and Sunday be a little easier on yourself. If you feel you have to eat that chicken parmesan over pasta, go for it, but Monday morning get right back on your clean five meals a day. Do this for a month. In the second month only go off the plan for two weekends. By the third month get on the plan full time. Using this method you'll really start to see fat shed from your body rapidly. This is the key.

Of course, the optimal plan is to simply start full time right away. If you do that you'll be wondering where that fat went in no time.

No matter what plan you choose you're going to see fat loss and that's what's going to make it easier for you. Remember don't worry about weight loss. Just keep stating your body's composition, and trust me: fat will begin to melt away.

Two things will alert you that you're reaching your goal. First, you will be very hungry an hour or so after a meal. Your metabolic rate has increased. Embrace this hunger and let it empower you. Let hunger be your friend. At that moment your body's metabolic rate is burning a ton of fat. Secondly, when you eat a meal, you begin to sweat. It usually happens to me at breakfast. I sit down to eat, my body recognizes the food, cranks up the metabolic rate and I break out in a sweat. You're just going to have to take this on faith: it's a good sweat. Try it and see.

❦ ❦ ❦

Let's take a look at breakfast. Besides being the start of the day, this will also be the hardest meal for most of us to become accustomed to the changes. This is where I'm going to take away some of your favorite foods, but if you stick with me they won't be your favorites much longer. Are you ready? Ok, we have to give up the fat, the dairy, the breads, and the fruit from this meal. No way? Sure there's a way. Suck it up and get over it. Besides, I won't expect you to do it all at once. Give up the dairy first or the fruit or the toast etc… Take a few weeks if you need it. And remember those berries. I'm going to let you have berries—a few of them.

What kills us with this meal is the bacon, sausage, bread, toast, egg yolks, fruit, juices, milk, cheese, the refined cereals. Basically everything you eat for breakfast right? Right.

Okay, but look at it from a different angle: You can have your eggs, but just the whites. I separate my egg yolks from the white by scooping them out of the bowl after I've cracked all the eggs. Or you can try the very good pasteurized pure egg white products sold in the market. It's expensive, but it does the job, so it's your choice. I won't take your cereal away, I'm just going to change it. From now on our complex carbohydrate is oatmeal, grits or cream of wheat—whichever you prefer. I prefer oatmeal. It's important to get Old Fashioned Oatmeal, not the quick kind. Why? Because the quick kind is ground up into finer particles. That's the company digesting it for you, so its absorbed more quickly causing a faster insulin spike—which we don't want. Also pass on the packets—you might as well eat a candy bar. The grits, cream of wheat or oatmeal must be made with good old fashion water. No milk! Add Equal or Splenda to your liking, with a small handful of berries. I like to sprinkle McCormick Cinnamon over the top. With me it has to be McCormick, because if it weren't my best friend, Dave—a McCormick's executive— would pull my boy off the pitcher's mound.

Your egg whites can be made any way you wish. I make an omelet with vegetables. Some people scramble them. One of my buddies simply drinks them down, the pasteurized type that is.

He says he doesn't have time to cook. If it meant eating raw egg whites I told him to get up a bit earlier because that is really nasty and dangerous. I don't advise it.

Along with fruit, bacon, sausage, juice, and toast, we have also eliminated butter and refined sugars from our breakfast table.

Drink water or coffee with Splenda or Equal and a splash of fat free milk, if you prefer.

If you're still hungry after the egg whites and oatmeal, consider a protein shake.

THE MR. MARYLAND COMPETITION:

As I told you I was two days away from the Mr. Maryland Competition. Well now it's here. I'm on a break between compulsories and the evening entertainment (individual routines). I'm competing in the Men's Open Light Heavy-Weight and the Masters over-40 group. Compared to the competition, I think I look pretty good. Do I think I'll be the next 2004 Mr. Maryland? Not a chance. The sanction that the Mr. Maryland falls under is called the NPC, the National Physique Committee. Unfortunately the NPC is the only sanction that I compete in which is not drug-tested. There are a lot of athletes here who are using supplements that I don't advocate or condone. It is fun, however, to be a natural bodybuilder and compete against others.

In my lectures I dedicate a short segment to time management. Some people have plenty of time, and don't have to worry about when we're going to fix all this food. I don't. Some of you don't either, so I'm going to tell those of you who have tight schedules how I get this stuff done. I'm not suggesting this is precisely the way you should do the cooking, I'm just using this as a point of departure. Take a good look at my method, then create your own.

For the rest of you this section will still have value as an illustration of one man's diet, and how the meals get balanced.

When I first started preparing food and eating right, I was fixing it the night before. For many of us this will be the fastest way to get tired, bored, and fall off the plan. For those of us without the time and/or inclination for every-night cook-offs, it's far better to use a couple of hours on a Saturday or Sunday (or whatever day you're free) and invest in some Tupperware. My norm is chicken breast, turkey breast, and tuna fish. Your turkey and chicken breast are simply dusted with whichever Ms. Dash's seasoning that you like the best. They have a ton so try them all. You can bake all of these dishes in the oven together to make the most of your time. While the meat cooks on one rack, I'll be baking four sweet potatoes and four regular potatoes on the other.

While these bake, I'll open three or four large cans of solid white albacore tuna packed in water. I strain the tuna and place it in a large Tupperware container. I'll add fat free mayo (and if you think you don't like fat free mayo, try it for a week; you'll forget what the bad stuff tastes like), chopped up celery, whatever spices suit your fancy and then mix it all up. Boom, you're done with your tuna salad. Into the fridge it goes. Kept at proper temperature, it stays fine for a week.

Not long after that I take out the baked chicken breasts. I cube or slice these, then put them into another large Tupperware container. Once again, I go with celery, fat free mayo and various spices. Any spices will do, but I live in Baltimore, so I only use McCormick.

By this time the self-timing thermometer in the turkey breast has popped out and my potatoes are just about done. I let the turkey cool before I cut it. Also it doesn't cut or cube as nicely when it's hot. I prepare the turkey just as I did the chicken, then I let the potatoes cool and cut them in half. I put these halves in individual baggies, then into a large Tupperware container which goes in the fridge.

This covers my twenty-one midday meals for the week.

In the evening when I'm preparing my dinner I'll set out four Tupperware containers. I'll take some of the veggies that will be used for my dinner salad and place them in three of the containers. I will also place some lettuce in these containers. I will then scoop out a big portion of tuna, turkey, and chicken salad into each of the three containers that have the veggies in them. In my fourth container I will place three potato halves. I'll eat one of these potatoes with each salad. I usually don't put anything extra on the tuna salad but feel free to put red wine vinegar, a little fat free dressing, a bit of salsa, a little Heinz 57, or possibly a little yellow or spicy mustard. If you do something like this it won't be long before you find yourself getting addicted to the lifestyle. Then you'll begin to say "Hey, I don't even really need the fat free mayo in my salad. I'll just eat the chicken on green veggies." Why will you say this? Because within two to three weeks of starting this new nutritional fitness program you're going to shed so much fat it will blow you away.

A brilliant man once said, "Try to enjoy food for its natural flavor." This is the way food is supposed to feel and taste in your mouth. In this country we try so hard to mask the natural taste of food that sometimes it is easy to forget what you are eating. Who was the man who had this simple, yet incisive view of food? You've probably heard of him. He came to this country with absolutely nothing, and became the world's greatest known bodybuilder. He worked his way to Hollywood stardom, married a Kennedy, and is now governor of California: Arnold Schwarzenegger. He is the epitome of the American Dream!

It's a lot of meals we're making here. We'll need them. We're going to spread them throughout the day, whether it be a work day or the weekend. I usually eat about every four hours, so this goes beyond the old three-square-meals-per-day. Just before I eat I'm usually so hungry that I'm getting a bit anxious. My staff will attest to that. Don't tell me you don't have time for these three meals during the workday. If you have time to go to the bathroom or take a coffee break, you have time for this.

But, you ask, is there anything else I can eat with these meals? Sure. These aren't the exact meals you have to eat. How creative a cook are you? I'll be getting into sauces and condiments later. That should stimulate the taste buds of the chefs out there.

If you've never thought much about cooking, this is the time to start. How much do you know about all the foods in the world? I've cut out a lot of them, but I've left in plenty. Just remember: lean protein, complex carbs, low fat. You build and operate your body off these. Think of all the things you can do with rice as long as you have a spice rack. Imagine the varieties of fish and chicken you can make with a shelf full of low-fat sauces. Look at all the ingredients you can have, and combine several into a marinade. And how does that same marinade taste over rice? Or even as a topping on the potato?

We'll also go into supplements. I'll go into these in detail later, but here and now you should understand that a supplement is just that! They are not a substitute for the whole diet, or even a real meal. One of my mentors, Mr. John Parrillo is in the supplement business, but he feels if your diet is not appropriate you should never take supplements. I am in complete agreement.

Back to our meals: Though we have covered the basic midday meals for the week, I don't want you to get in a rut. Don't always eat potatoes. I do it because I love them, but feel free to substitute some delicious steamed brown rice. If you have a rice steamer that makes it easy. If not boil a big pot of rice on Sunday and scoop it out as you go along throughout the week. The same thing goes for black beans, pinto beans, black eyed peas, fresh corn, etc… These are a lot of starchy carbohydrates. Mix it up and have fun with it but take a small portion of starchy carbohydrate with every lean protein meal.

Mix up your veggies as well. Like I said: If it's green, eat it. Enjoy the natural flavor of raw, crisp vegetables with your lean protein salad.

With proteins I'll require some restrictions on substitutes: stay with our white, lean protein sources (i.e. chicken, fish and turkey). The fish portion doesn't always have to be tuna. I simply find tuna easy to manage (i.e. from the can to the Tupperware). If you're game for cooking a couple of pounds of cod or salmon or for that matter any fish and spread it out all week have at it.

I placed first in the Masters over-40 division of the NPC Maryland State Championships. I guess that makes me Mr. "Old Fogie" Maryland for 2004. I also scored a second place finish in the men's' open light heavy weight division. My loss was to a man half my age who had about ten extra pounds of muscle to his physique.

A young bodybuilder who had been "dieting down" for this show for about twelve weeks reported to me that he had eaten no other protein source but cod fish six times per day for the last six weeks. I thought this was a little extreme. "Dieting down" in bodybuilding is a grueling regimen where one has to virtually eliminate complex carbohydrates and fats from one's diet for an extended period of time, while maintaining a high level of cardiovascular training, and strength training with weights. This forces the body into a catabolic state where it attempts to use all of the body's fat stores for energy. The bodybuilder maintains a high protein intake with hopes of not burning lean muscle tissue. Unfortunately these guys always burn lean tissue. I've also seen people go through dermatitis (Their skin peels off) and alopecia (loss of hair) from this kind of regimen.

When these poor, sick, starving kids ask me how long I diet down, I tell them I don't. They want to know how I, at forty-two, can compete with the younger men. I tell them it's my lifestyle. I follow the "Hands of Time" philosophy 24/7, 365 days a year. They're amazed, but they shouldn't be.

After the competition, when every one else was talking about binging on pizza and beer, I chuckled. I had no more desire to drown my second place finish in a pizza then I did fly to the moon. Instead I enjoyed a couple of cold Miller Lites, a treat I hadn't allowed myself in a few weeks.

Okay, we've covered the majority of the day's nutritional intake. We're left with the final meal. This is the meal where most people make their worst mistakes: late night carbs. Unfortunately I eat very late by American standards, and I don't suggest you imitate me in this respect.

Nonetheless, I'm the one advocating this diet, so for those of you who work late like I do, let me describe what I do: I'll arrive home between 7 and 8 p.m. While the kids hit the shower, I hit the gym. Fifteen or twenty minutes is all that's necessary. I'll strength train for a few minutes. By this time its 8:45 or 9 p.m. Not a great time to start dinner right?

A lot of you would tell me: I already ate my breakfast and three midday meals, so why not skip the night meal? Wouldn't that help with the fat loss? No! Get out of this mindset. Although the metabolic rate is slowest during sleep, this meal gives us the potential for greatest fat loss. The key is to eat food that virtually can't be turned to fat.

Though my late night dinner usually falls between 9:30 and 10 p.m., it is clean. It consists of a lean protein source and fibrous carbohydrates. I take no fats (except what's associated with the chicken, turkey, or fish) or starchy carbohydrates at this meal.

At this meal I eat either turkey, fish, chicken, steak (lean) or an occasional crabcake. Whatever main course, I have it broiled, baked, or at best pan-seared.

The fibrous carbohydrates are two-fold. I always like to have a salad. I prefer such food as romaine lettuce, tomatoes, mushrooms, cucumbers, and Vidalia onions if they're in season. If not I go for the sweet white onions, lots and lots of onions. My wife hates to kiss me! I also have steamed veggies. I almost always have asparagus; sometimes I'll add broccoli and cauliflower. These go into a microwave dish with some water and a bit of Mrs. Dash. In two minutes they're done.

How do I dress up the main course? This is critical. If you had to eat nothing but plain turkey, fish, chicken, or shellfish all the time, this would be terrible. So what are we going to do? I'm not a chef, and this is not a recipe book, but I'm going to tell you your options and let you have at it. There are a lot of sauces and toppings that make my food exciting.

Sometimes I use barbeque sauce. The one I select is called Stubbs'. There's no fat and only three grams of sugar. All the rest of the barbeque sauces out there are loaded with sugar. Trust me I've searched. For most of us the original Stubbs' will be spicy enough. Then there's *Newman's Own* salsa –no fat and only one gram of sugar. Seriously how can you go wrong? Salsa is great over anything. I put it on both turkey breast cutlets or make Mexican turkey burgers. It's just as good over chicken breast. Salsa is salsa, usually no fat and low sugar. The thing to watch out for is the sodium count. Newman's Own is moderate and that's why I buy it.

Another favorite is *Healthy Choice* tomato/pasta sauce (it comes in all varieties). There's no fat and only seven grams of sugar. It's been my finding over the years that if you can keep your fat grams in your sauces under five grams and your sugar grams under ten, you're doing great.

Back to the pasta sauce. I like Chicken Parm. The chicken is baked or broiled as indicated and then smothered with *Healthy Choice* pasta sauce. The pasta sauce is then sprinkled heavily with fat free Parmesan cheese grated topping and allowed to broil another few minutes. I swear you'll never be able to tell the difference between this and your favorite Italian restaurant.

One topping I often choose is *Heinz 57* sauce. No fat and only a few grams of sugar. Trust me it's not just for steak. It will dress up any of your lean protein meals.

Kudos to *Kraft* fat-free salad dressings. They're great! They have many varieties and none have any fat! What you do have to note is the sugar content. I like the Bleu Cheese. It's great on a steak as well as chicken or turkey. Obviously it works well on your salad veggies but I'm unorthodox, and use it as a dip to enhance Maryland Crabcakes! Try it, it's great! The Ranch is also very good.

Kraft fat-free sliced American or cheddar cheese – what a treat. One gram of sugar and zero grams of fat. At 250 mg the sodium is a bit high, so don't eat too many slices. I enjoy these mixed with my omelet in the AM or over ground turkey breast burgers in the evening. Try a melted piece of cheddar over the turkey salsa burger for dinner. I bet you have to eat a second burger! I also enjoy this cheese as a munchie during preparation of dinner. I'll take a slice, pour brown mustard on it then snack.

Which brings me to mustards and ketchups. Surprisingly they're not bad at all. Read the labels but the mustards routinely have no fat and no sugar. Sodium concentrations are also normally good, especially with the yellow mustards. Brown mustards also have low to no fat and sugars but their sodium concentrations are a bit high. Ketchups are surprisingly the same on fat and sodium, but some have higher sugar. Most are no fat and less than five grams of sugar. I swear, I put mustard on anything. Obviously I use it on my turkey and tuna and chicken that I eat during the day, but I'm also prone to use it on veggies at night. I'll snack on carrots and mustard, celery and mustard, fat free cheese and mustard, and broccoli and mustard. I'm a mustard-aholic!

Look out for low-fat peanut butter. You're sailing into uncharted waters. Here we move up in fat and sugar. But what a treat, spread lightly on a cracker. I can't think of anything better. I'm not giving the green light on this as an everyday thing, but once or twice a week is okay–a treat! Just don't make a meal of it.

Could life be complete if we didn't have crackers? Yes, trust me you'll live—just like I do every day. But if you must treat on the peanut butter and crackers, the most wholesome and nutritious crackers on the market are Wasa crackers. Wasa crackers are truly whole grain, no fat, no sugars, and only a few simple carbs. They're also very low in sodium. Still they are crackers, a simple carbohydrate no matter how you cut it. So remember there is no law that says peanut butter must be spread on anything. Have you tried it right from the jar? That's my preferred technique. Make sure you change spoons if you double dip.

I'm clearly not a chef and this is clearly not a cookbook. You have to use your imagination. I told you this would be a huge change in your diet, a huge lifestyle change, and I told you it wouldn't be easy. But again if you stick with it, it will alter your entire being. Nutrition is everything. Remember those words. You are what you eat. This is gospel!

Chapter V

MEASURE BY MEASURE

This chapter is all about the math behind the madness. It's a close examination of nutrition and fat loss. Let's start with an evaluation of the body's composition and how to monitor it. Body composition testing can be performed a number of different ways. I find skin calipers to be the most efficient and accurate way to test body composition. Other techniques are buoyancy and water displacement in a pool designed for body fat measurement, and electronic scales which detect the percentage of body fat. I find this last method to be very unreliable and inaccurate. I've been told that the pool of water is the most accurate method for measurement but how many people have the opportunity to be measured in this fashion? Skin fold calipers are convenient and accurate. In less than five minutes you can calculate your body's fat composition.

We are measuring the body's percentage of lean mass and fat mass out of the total body weight. The body's lean mass consists of muscle, bone, and organ tissue. Body composition testing is an accurate measure of the body's fluctuation in total weight based on the changing percentages of these masses.

> When I'm going into competition people always ask me what I'll weigh at check-in. I always put light heavy-weight on the applications because usually that is where I will be: between 180 and 195 pounds. I know that right now, though I haven't stepped on a scale in six months. This is the attitude I want you to empower. To do it, you'll have to start with a body weight measurement then continue body stating. You will weigh yourself once a week only; other than this STAY OFF THAT SCALE! What you weigh does not matter! It's all based around your fat composition. That's all. What is your fat composition and how do you look when standing in front of that full-length mirror? That's what you should worry about.

A skin fold caliper is a spring-loaded device, which measures the thickness of a fold of skin with its underlying layer of fat. The spring exerts a specific force on the jaws of the caliper and a scale in millimeters is used to measure the thickness of the skin fold. By measuring nine specific locations on the body we can calculate that person's body composition. There are three things to keep in mind when performing body stat calculations. Measure as close to the designated area as you can. In that area, try to measure the location with the most fatty tissue. If you measure a lean pinch from that area you get an inaccurate composition and the person won't notice a decrease in fat composition as they begin to lose fat. Lastly always measure the same spot. Be as accurate as you can about this.

If you're right handed hold the caliper in your right hand. Pull out a fold of skin from the location. Hold the calipers a half inch from your fingers. Completely release the jaw of the calipers on the skin fold. Don't release the skin fold from your opposite hand. Once released, the jaw will creep a bit on the skin fold. This creeping represents fluid being squeezed from the underlying subcutaneous tissue. The creep will stop, then you should measure the number of millimeters at that fold and record accordingly on your stat sheet. Your body stating sheet should have weekly readings recorded next to one another to measure your progress.

There are nine spots on the body to measure:

1.**Pectoral** – Skin fold should be pulled out horizontally about one inch below the collar bone at the mid-muscle mark. Stay off of breast tissue in females, stay on skin and directly over muscle.

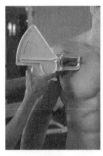

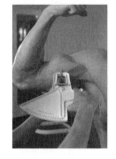

2.**Subscapular** – Skin fold should be measured in a vertical direction. The middle of the scapula or shoulder blade is located and the skin fold is pinched one inch towards the spine.

3.**Biceps** – Skin fold is measured in a vertical direction. The pinch should be in the mid-muscle area.

4.**Triceps** – Skin fold is measured in a vertical direction. The pinch should be at the bottom of an innermost portion of the tricep muscle.

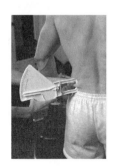

5.**Kidney** – Skin fold should be measured in a horizontal direction. Locate the indentation above the gluteus muscle along the waist. Measure up two inches and out two inches directly over the kidneys

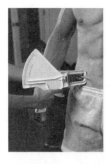

6.**Suprailiac** – Skin fold is measured in a horizontal direction. The pinch is taken half way between the navel and the crest of the iliac bone (hip).

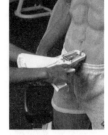

7.**Abdominals** – Skin fold is measured in a vertical direction. The pinch is taken one inch lateral to and one inch below the navel.

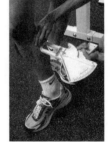

8.**Quadriceps** – Skin fold is measured in a vertical direction. Measure right in the middle of the quadriceps muscle on the front.

9.**Medial Calf** – Skin fold is measured in a vertical direction. The pinch is taken on the inner side of the muscle in the middle.

These measurements are recorded on a BodyStat sheet.

These numbers are your tools for determining your body composition. To do that, you add the nine measurements and divide by your weight. This gives the ratio of body fat to body weight. This number is multiplied by .27 to get the percentage of body fat. Multiply the body weight by the percentage of body fat to get the pounds of body fat. Subtract the pounds of body fat from the body weight to calculate the pounds of lean mass.

To analyze the data you compare the numbers to the previous week. From this information, you plan your appropriate course of action.

BodyStat Sheet   Name_____

Date						
Pec (--)						
Subscapular (I)						
Bicep (I)						
Tricep (I)						
Kidney (--)						
Suprailiac (--)						
Abdominals (I)						
Quadricep (I)						
Medial Calf (I)						
Total						
Bodyweight						
Total/Bodyweight						
Total/Bodyweight x .27 = % Bodyfat						
%Bodyfat x Bodyweight = lbs. Bodyfat						
Change in Bodyfat from Previous Week						
Bodyweight - lbs. Bodyfat = lbs. Lean Mass						
Change in Lean Mass from Previous Week						

Parrillo Performance

-51-

Generally speaking, fit and athletic males should have a body fat percentage between 12% and 15 %. Athletic females should be between 18% to 20 %. If the body fat compositions are higher that's no problem. That's what we're addressing with the Hands of Time lifestyle. Very rapidly you will begin to shed fat and not only reach these goals, but go well beyond, if that is what you choose.

If your initial measurements are high you want to try and shed one half a pound of body fat per week until you get to your suggested levels. Ways to do this are to increase our aerobic exercises to boost metabolism, make sure that dietary fats don't exceed 5% of your over all caloric intake and decrease your complex carbohydrates and begin to consume more fibrous carbohydrates.

Examples of changes that can accrue from week to week are given below:

If you lose lean mass you are clearly not eating enough. You need to increase your nutritional consumption of protein, complex carbohydrates, fibrous carbohydrates, and fats in the appropriate percentages.

If you gain mass and maintain your fat you may need to increase your caloric intake by 150 to 350 calories per day to maintain the new lean muscle tissue while also increasing your cardiovascular aerobic exercises to burn more fat.

If you gain lean mass and lose fat this is great! You're on the right path. Continue your nutritional intake and exercise regime as you are, but monitor weekly to make sure you're nutritional intake doesn't become too deficient for the new lean tissue.

If you gain mass and gain fat this is okay as long as you stay in that athletic range. If the fat percentage increases beyond this, increase your aerobics a bit or take a good look at your diet. Are you taking in too many fatty or processed foods? Do you need to decrease your complex carbohydrates a bit?

If you maintain mass and maintain fat you've hit a plateau. You need to do something different. Increase your lean protein a little and train a bit heavier or longer. Increase your cardiovascular exercises.

If you maintain your mass and lose fat as some women like to do: Great! Again you're on the right track. Remember though, you can't gain lean mass in this state. You may need to increase your caloric intake by 150 to 350 calories per day to begin to gain mass.

Calipers for measuring body fat composition can easily be ordered through Parrillo Nutritional products at 1-800-344-3404.

We've been talking a lot about caloric intake, the types of foods to eat, how to change or increase your calories to affect your fat loss, etc... You obviously need a baseline from which to start. Our lean protein should make up about 45-55% of our diet. Complex and fibrous carbohydrates should make up about 35-45% of our diets and fats should make up about 5-10% of our nutritional intake.

By calculating the Specific Dynamic Action of our bodies we can determine what our optimum number of calories should be in a 24-hour period.

The Specific Dynamic Action (SDA) equals our Basal Metabolic Rate (BMR) plus our Voluntary Muscular Activity (VMA). Our BMR is our body weight in kilograms-times-24. Our VMA equals our BMR times our activity level (i.e. .50 for a sedentary person, .75 for a very active individual and 1.0 for an extreme athlete).

The formula looks like this:

$$SDA = BMR + VMA$$
$$BMR = BW(kg) \times 24$$
$$VMA = BMR \times (.50, .75, \text{ or } 1.0)$$

Please note: your body weight in kg can be calculated by dividing your body weight in pounds by 2.2.

How do you figure the number of calories in your food? You buy a food counting book. There are a number of them on the market but I find the easiest one to read is the *CTN Series of Food Counts*. Ms. Corinne T. Netzer has devoted her life to figuring out exactly the number of calories, grams of protein, carbohydrates, fats and sugar in all the foods we eat.

And lastly how do we know how much food to eat and whether our percentages are appropriate? That's easy. Buy a food scale. Ms. Netzer will tell you how many calories are in a six-ounce chicken breast or eight ounces of tuna. You simply use these numbers to figure out what your percentages are to formulate your diet. Do the math.

Food scales are inexpensive and available at any kitchen store, or from John Parrillo. Sounds like a lot of work to simply eat right? Like any other task it will quickly become habit whenever you eat a new food. You'll only have to weigh the regular foods in your diet once or twice. That will tell you what size your portions should be and you can set your scale aside until the next time you introduce a new food to your diet. Also you will occasionally need it to increase or decrease a specific nutritional component, for instance: decreasing your calories of complex carbohydrates because of continued fat gain.

Chapter VI

THE CHEAT MEAL

Now we arrive at The Cheat Meal. I was going to go for the Guinness World Record for the shortest chapter ever, and simply write: "EAT ANYTHING." But then I realized I had better explain.

The cheat meal is where you reward yourself. You've busted your ass all week long working out and eating 35 –42 clean meals and this is where you get a break! I look forward to my cheat meal all week long starting on Sunday morning. You guessed it: I normally eat my cheat meal on Saturday night.

What do I typically eat? The sky's the limit. I eat and drink whatever I want. When my wife and I get a babysitter, we'll go out to dinner, start with cocktails, have an appetizer, a salad, an entrée and then coffee with possibly an after dinner drink. On the other hand, if we're with the kids, we'll usually do pizza and beer, or Mexican and beer. I deserve it. I'm not a big dessert fan but if you are, go for it! You deserve it!

I eat this way even before a competition. Granted I may skip the alcohol or ask to have my steak cooked clean with no salt or marinade, but I don't have to.

How does that sound? Good? I thought so. Does this bring back some perspective? We're all human beings, and from time to time, we want to eat exactly what we feel like eating.

But (and this is a big "but") after your cheat meal, I want you right back on that clean tight nutritional intake every three-to-four hours for another week.

Chapter VII

SUPPLEMENTS

Any book written about nutrition, fitness and training would be remiss without a section on supplements. Let's be clear: The person who initially taught me how to eat trained me for a year without letting me eat supplements. Why? Because supplements are just that—supplements. They're a way to increase your caloric intake of specific nutrients which your body will use to gain lean mass and shed fat. But this is not what the supplement companies would have you believe. They'll say that if you try their new pill, shake, or bar you're going to become Superman. It doesn't work that way.

I recently cancelled my subscription to *Muscle and Fitness* magazine. I got tired of seeing all those supplement ads where scarcely-clad babes cluster around huge drug-induced bodybuilders. They tell us: take this pill, gain fifty pounds of solid muscle, and watch the gals come-a-running. What a joke!

The worst offender is the meal replacement supplement. Whether it's a shake or a bar, there's no such thing as a replacement for a good, nutritious meal. None! You've got to eat real, clean food. That's the only path to shedding fat and growing muscle.

Only when you've disciplined yourself to eating clean can you begin to supplement your diet to increase your calories and give your body the extra energy or protein that it needs to grow.

I'll discuss a few supplements here. These are the only ones you'll ever need, once your diet and exercise regime is squared away. They are the ones that work.

CREATINE MONOHYDRATE

Creatine is a recent supplement which hit the bodybuilding world like a ton of bricks. Why? Because it works! Creatine Monohydrate if taken correctly—loading dose followed by a maintenance dose—can actually add five-to-fifteen pounds of lean mass to your body in less than a month. A miracle drug, right? Wrong. The weight gain is all water and I'll tell you why.

Cellular energy comes from a molecule called ATP (adenosine triphosphate). It's formed from the chemical energy in food. The body has only a small store of ATP. When the ATP is used for energy, Creatine Phosphate comes in to re-form more ATP. In weight lifting the ATP and the CP are generally used up in a minute or so. This is why our muscles fail at the end of a long set of lifting exercises. However, in aerobic exercises (long distance running and biking) the body can continue to produce ATP and CP because the exercise is of lower intensity and can continue almost indefinitely.

Creatine Monohydrate as opposed to Creatine Phosphate crosses the intestinal layer, then is absorbed into the muscle cell and acts as another source of energy for the muscle cell to produce more ATP and work harder and longer.

Creatine attracts water, so once it's in the muscle cell, water follows, swelling the muscle. This isn't true muscle growth.

Remember, Creatine does not increase muscle protein. This is critical. Then what's this about muscle growth? Creatine provides the muscle with more energy and power allowing the muscle to work harder and longer. This in combination with a good clean healthy diet high in lean protein and complex carbohydrates will stimulate the muscle tissue to hypertrophy (grow). While Creatine does not create new muscles, if used correctly it can create the conditions for new muscle growth.

But this initial weight gain in lean tissue mass comes with a price. All that increase in water has a tendency to make you flat looking. In other words, you don't get the muscle definition that a person would have if they are not taking Creatine. However, if taken correctly it does have merit and will work.

When I used to take Creatine (I don't anymore) I found that it gave me prostatitis. Don't ask me how or why, but when I stopped taking it the prostatitis went away. This is the reason I choose not to take Creatine Monohydrate. Keep this in mind if the same thing happens to you.

MEDIUM CHAIN TRIGLYCERIDE OIL

Medium Chain Triglyceride Oil (MCT Oil) is a distilled and refined product from coconut oil. It is cholesterol-free, and doesn't have the adverse qualities of regular coconut oil. MCT has a much shorter molecule than conventional oils. It is rapidly oxidized by the body having little tendency to be stored as fat.

Study after study of MCT oils show that this product boosts the body's thermogenesis effect (the production of body heat from the burning of food). It increases your body's ability to burn fat.

MCT oil is rapidly absorbed by the gastrointestinal tract and into the hepatic portal system. It is transported to the liver and converted into ketones. Ketones enter the blood stream and can be used as fuel when glycogen stores are low. This use as energy gives the MCT oil the ability to spare muscle protein from being broken down and used as energy.

Also when triglycerides like MCT oil are present, the enzymes in the liver that convert glucose into fat are less active. In other words MCT oil not only helps burn fat but also helps avoid production and storage of new fat.

MCT oil has to be introduced to the body very slowly, because it may initially cause abdominal cramping and diarrhea. MCT oil is a great product. I highly advocate it. I use it mostly on the off-season when I'm trying to put on a few extra pounds of muscle. However, if I take it too close to a competition, I feel a little smoother, and not quite as shredded. I usually discontinue MCT oils four weeks prior to a competition.

WHEY PROTEIN

Whey Protein is in most of the protein supplements on the market today. Whey is a component of milk. It is separated from milk to make cheese and other dairy products.

For those of you who have milk allergies there are products on the market today made from egg protein and soy protein, but I will only address whey protein here.

Whey protein has a high concentration of the Branch Chain Amino Acids (BCAAs). These—especially Leucine—play a significant role in muscle protein synthesis. Additionally Leucine plays a large role in facilitating loss of subcutaneous and visceral (deep) fat loss.

Whey protein is an excellent recovery nutrient. Studies have shown that whey protein taken after exercise promotes glycogen re-synthesis. In other words whey protein helps you rebuild your muscle energy quicker so you can work out harder and see faster gains in lean mass and losses of fat.

I personally take a whey protein shake with four out of my five daily meals. It provides me some additional calories and gets me to the 1.0-1.5 grams of protein per pound of body weight that I shoot for.

CARBOHYDRATE SUPPLEMENTS

Carbohydrate supplements come in a number of forms. I choose to eat bars, but shakes are available. Remember: these shakes are to be made with water, not milk!

The body can only store about 600 grams of glycogen. It's stored mostly in our muscles and some in the liver. As the glycogen is used up during exercise, the body reserves get low. The muscle glycogen is used first, then the liver converts the glycogen to glucose and releases it to the bloodstream. When it's gone it's gone. The point of muscle fatigue is the point of glycogen depletion. Also with glycogen depletion, fat and muscle are sometimes used as energy sources. Fat is a great energy source but muscle breakdown for energy is prohibited in the "Hands of Time" lifestyle.

Every individual has their own carbohydrate requirements. Obviously aerobic athletes require a lot more carbohydrates then weight lifters. Regardless of when we train we must replenish our carbohydrate stores. We will do this with complex carbohydrate foods and a carbohydrate supplement if necessary.

I try to shoot for around 250 – 300 grams of complex carbohydrates per day to avoid glycogen depletion. To supplement my diet I choose an energy bar about three times per day with my meals.

You have to be very careful with the labels of these products because simple sugars hide under different names. Be careful about sugar alcohols. I try to stay with products that contain Dextrins as slow-release starches. I know these are not sugars.

Mr. John Parrillo has an excellent selection of all of these products. His quality control is superb and his products taste great. Trust me, I've tried a ton of products out there and Parrillo products are the finest available, bar none.

John's clients are mostly athletes, and when he's finished with them they are usually champion athletes. At this writing, John and I are working together in an effort to produce supplements to be used by the average person—the non-athlete.

EPHEDRA

Ephedra is a supplement which was recently banned by the FDA. I used to take it about a week before a show to get that little extra bit of subcutaneous fat off. It was a dangerous product, and I'm glad it is off the market. Ephedra was the subject of concern in a number of deaths of both amateur and professional athletes, including twenty-three-year-old pitcher, Steve Bechler of the Baltimore Orioles. Ephedra increased one's overall basal metabolic rate. It also increased both blood pressure and your heart rate. If you've ever taken it, you know how it gives you that two-pots-of-coffee, hair-on-end feeling which is always uncomfortable. Back when I used it I always felt wiped out when a show was over—what a withdrawal. I would feel lethargic and run down for about a week.

I assumed it was a safe supplement taken as directed, but people often stretch the directions on pills. There's the feeling that if one pill is good then two pills must be better. I believe this is why so many people got sick and died from this stuff. I'm glad it's off the market.

This practice still goes on. When I was at the Mr. Maryland competition I heard a few guys saying they had purchased pseudophedrine, the active ingredient in a decongestant medication sold over the counter. They were doubling and tripling the normal dosage to get that increased metabolic, fat-burning quality. Don't take these chances with your body. The return is not worth the risk.

Chapter VIII

The Real Work—Cardio

Can you believe it! We finally made it to exercise. You knew it was coming. Or did you hope I'd never get there? Our next two chapters are dedicated to training. We'll begin with cardiovascular training, while in the second, we'll cover strength or resistance training. I put cardio first because it is the most beneficial in overall day-to-day health. I will emphasize resistance training slightly more in terms of physique and fat loss, but even here cardio training is important. Both are critical to our quest.

I've told you that diet and nutrition are 80% of the ball game. I mean it. If you stick to the diet I've outlined, you will recognize huge amounts of fat loss, even if you choose not to train.

So why kill ourselves? Why bother to work up a sweat three or four times per week, for forty minutes each time if we don't need to. Here's why: You want to see fat loss right? Combining cardiovascular and resistance exercises with the diet will dramatically speed up the changes you will see. If you do the cardiovascular exercise and resistance training along with the diet, you will see results within ten days. With the diet alone you won't begin to notice changes for six to eight weeks. Eight weeks of diet in concert with cardio and strength training will virtually transform your existence, and at twelve weeks the metamorphosis will be complete. The change in your health and physique will be incredible.

If you think: "Well, I just don't like exercise, so I'll skip the training," think again. Those months before you see results will be long ones indeed. Go ahead if you think you can, and are that dedicated to your standing as a couch potato, but with the training comes reinforcement for your self-discipline, and that is the key component for most of us. If you are doing the training, it is at three months that the program bows out, and you are completely on your own.

I already talked about the need for self-discipline. It's true at the start, and even more true in those first few weeks. At three months, it will be entirely up to you and the discipline you find within yourself. The results of the program may give you impetus, but it's your responsibility to use it.

I can't emphasize this enough. When you reach this point you may do what you wish. You can fall off the nutritional plan and stop exercising and become fat again or you can take it to the next level. My gut feeling is that most of you will do the latter. Why? Because once you've learned how to eat and exercise, it becomes entrenched in your lifestyle. Soon, you won't even remember how you ate before. In addition your exercise regimen has taken you to a high level of health, and produced a physique that you won't want to give up. When temptation comes you won't risk it.

At three months your new nutrition and exercise plan has significantly changed things. Guess what? You're healthy! How long has it been? You're eating clean, exercising hard and feeling better than you ever did before. I have seen people who have been able to safely discontinue blood pressure medication, oral hypoglycemic (diabetes) medication, high cholesterol medication and arthritic medication simply by following the Hands of Time lifestyle. I have one friend who had suffered from Raynaud's Syndrome for years. After starting my program, this completely disappeared to the amazement of my friend and her physician.

Let's start with cardiovascular training – what it is and why it is so important in our lives. Cardiovascular training is something you've probably heard of plenty of times under another name: aerobic exercise.

One question I often get in my seminars is: Which type of cardiovascular exercise is best? I love this question because the answer is so simple: IT DOESN'T MATTER! What do you like? Jogging, speed walking, swimming, racquetball, elliptical trainer, jumping rope... IT DOESN'T MATTER! What does matter is that you get it done.

The American College of Sports Medicine recommends twenty-to-thirty minutes of cardiovascular training at least three times per week where you reach your Target Heart Rate (THR). What is THR? It is an elevation in heart rate to a specific level based upon your age and level of conditioning. When your cardiovascular exercise is vigorous enough to take your heart rate to this level it provides benefits to your overall systemic health. You can determine your THR by using The Karvonen Formula below:

(220 - age) - resting-heart-rate x training-intensity [.50 (50%, light) or .60 (60%, moderate) or possibly .80 (80%, intense)] + resting heart rate=THR

So, if our sample person is 45 and has a resting heart rate of 70 and a moderate level of training intensity (.60), then it would be:

220 - 45 = 175, then 175 - 70 = 105, then 105 x .60 = 63, then 63 + 70 = 133.
Our sample person will have a THR of 133.

Your training intensity is the real variable here. How conditioned are you? Are you an athlete or a couch potato? (If you're a couch potato you might as well admit it; after all, you're the person who's going to benefit most from this plan.) If you exercise little or not at all the training intensity will have to be low.

As you start the program it's best to consult your doctor. I'll go into this in more detail later, but one thing you'll want to go into is training intensity. It will depend on your pre-program history and physical exam. It's usually best to start at about 40% - to - 50 %. Plug these numbers in to come up with a THR and see how you do on your first week of cardio. If you can't sustain this THR then slow down. You'll get there. Just take your time. As I've been telling you: you have the rest of your life. You'll see it come, and once you do, you'll be that much happier.

How do you measure your heart rate to see if you've reached your THR? There are a ton of automated devices that hook to your chest, head, or wrist. The device will monitor your heart rate while you do your cardio. Most institutional cardio machines (such as those in gyms and fitness centers) monitor this for you. All you do is grab a handle and the machine will tell you your pulse rate. Easy as that.

If you need to take the approach of strict measurement, buy a monitoring device.Or you can do as I do, and use The Sweat Rule. When I'm finished my cardio training I'm usually dripping wet. This way I know I've gone beyond what is necessary to stimulate my metabolic rate and burn fat.

So now, we're back to hard work. Cardio training is not easy. If it were everyone would do it, and everyone would be svelte and beautiful or handsome. Remember we live in the fattest country in the world. We Americans can get pretty lazy when it comes to exercise. It takes effort to stay healthy and lean, and when it comes to physical exertion most of us neglect it. We'll sit at a desk and work hard at our jobs all day, but we avoid physical work of all kinds.

I'm a bodybuilder, and from that viewpoint I'm about to commit heresy: At competitions I'm often questioned how I stay so lean at forty-two years of age. When this old man tells the young guys he was out drinking vodka and eating prime rib the weekend before the show, they get bent out of shape. When I go on the stage and beat them, they don't believe it.

So how can it be? Let's begin with the fact that I'm a little nuts. Most bodybuilders concentrate on Size, Size, Size: growing muscles big and thick. That's never been my goal. My only thought is to come in more conditioned than anyone else—usually, I do. Unfortunately, I sometimes lose to the bigger bodybuilder. Clearly mass and size is a big criteria in judging. And you know what? That's okay!

But these guys keep their cardiovascular training to a minimum. They're scared that they're going to lose lean mass. Most of them do little or no cardiovascular training in the offseason, but they do it three-to-four times per week during season.

I, the nutcase, do cardiovascular training seven days a week, 365 days per year. I don't expect you to do this. If you don't do it now, please don't start! It will burn you out and make you bored and tired of the program. To me there's nothing better than pulling on some sweats or shorts and doing a run at five a.m. I swear to God, this is like heaven.

Running down the road in the dark or at the crack of dawn, no one but the deer bounding through the fields, is the most pleasant thing in the world. No cars, lights, or any of the hustle and bustle of the later hours. It's quiet time to think and reflect and plan. I'm not suggesting that this is your thing, but find a method of cardiovascular training that you can learn to enjoy. Cardio and your new diet plan are your keys to metabolic increase and fat loss.

In my lectures and educational video, I explain that the only equipment necessary in our quest for ultimate health and a perfect physique is a pair of adjustable dumbbells, an adjustable bench, a body fat caliper, and a pair of running shoes. Let me suggest a cardio machine as well. Why? Because on the 7th of February when it's 14°F with six inches of snow on the ground, the last thing you want to do is pull on your running shoes and head outside. As

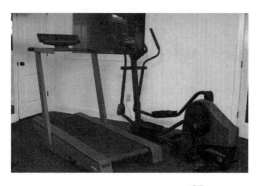

crazy as I am, I don't do it, but I don't skip my cardio that day either. No can do.

Instead I go to my basement and get on the treadmill or elliptical machine for a half hour. I can work up a good clean sweat on either of these machines. Many of you have a cardio machine at home. It's probably suffering from disuse. Any machine will do. Just stop using it as a clothes hanger, dust it off, oil it and have at it.

Now for one of the most important tricks. If you haven't heard anything I've talked about at all in the book, listen now. When do you do your cardiovascular training? There's only one best time during the day: First thing in the morning. And I mean FIRST, before you do anything else. Don't complain that you have too much to do: breakfast, shower, makeup, kids, school, etc. I do all these things too—with the exception of make-up! Get up a half hour earlier then you normally do. Get it done! If that means going to bed a half hour earlier, so be it. Remember, you are changing your life. With everything else that you're going to change, getting up a bit earlier to do your cardio will be the easy part.

I often see people running in the evening or afternoon. They're sweating in the day's heat and getting a super cardiovascular workout. God bless them, but what they don't understand is that they have already missed the prime opportunity to increase their metabolic rates for the entire day and stimulate their bodies to burn fat for the entire day. Why? I'll tell you.

At no time during the day are you more hypoglycemic (low blood sugar) than when you wake up in the morning. You've fasted all night and all those meals you've eaten the day before have your metabolic rate racing so fast that you've burned up everything in your system during the night's sleep. To use this to your advantage, you must wake up, pull on your shorts and shoes and do your cardio.

We have three compartments of energy in our bodies: the blood, the muscles and the liver. Within seven-to-ten minutes, the body uses up all the blood-borne glucose. Within the next seven-to-ten minutes the muscles convert their stored glycogen into glucose which they use for energy. In the next seven-to-ten minutes, the muscles are emptied and your body goes to its last energy supply. The liver stores of glycogen are then converted to glucose and dumped into the bloodstream for energy.

Since you started your moderate-to-intense cardiovascular exercise (to THR), twenty-to-thirty minutes have lapsed, and you're literally out of gas. You have no more energy to burn for your exercise, stored or otherwise.

So, what happens? You aren't collapsing on the street or the treadmill, I hope. No. Your will power and newfound discipline take you beyond that twenty-minute limit. At this point you are producing energy through a process known as gluconeogenesis: the production of glucose (energy) from non-carbohydrate sources. In other words, the body goes to its easiest store for energy: FAT. Fat is now mobilized, broken down, and converted to glucose. This is how you lose fat, plain and simple.

In *Chapter One* we talked about the amount of time you put into training. We said forty minutes per day, three-to-four days per week. You should break this forty minutes into 20 minutes of cardiovascular training to THR, and 20 minutes of strength training three-to-four times per week. If you really want to accelerate your fat loss increase your cardio training to thirty or forty minutes. The results will be unbelievable. This is really where you get into intense fat burning.

As a maintenance level of cardiovascular training I'll do twenty-to-thirty minutes a day. Again I'm not asking you to do this. Don't do anything extra that will burn you out on the program. I enjoy staying at 7 %-or-less body fat off season and at 5-6 % on season. There is absolutely no reason you need to stay this lean unless you want to. If you do, join me, and step it up. Otherwise keep it basic.

At my lectures I'm always faced with the issue that its impossible for everyone to do their cardiovascular training in the morning, *i.e.* single moms with kids, graveyard shift workers, people who leave for work at four a.m., etc. In these cases I explain there is another time AFTER your strength training. All too often I hear: "My personal trainer told me to do twenty minutes of cardiovascular exercise prior to strength training as a warm up." This is terrible advice! The only warm-up you need to strength train is a good stretch routine, which I'll discuss in the next chapter. Never do cardio prior to lifting. Never! You're burning up all that precious glucose and glycogen that you'll need in your muscles to be strong for your strength training.

If you absolutely can't do your cardio in the morning, do it after your strength training. At that point, you've burned up a lot of your glucose and glycogen while you were tearing down your muscle fibers doing your strength training. Your body is depleted of glucose and glycogen and this is the time to do your twenty-or-thirty minutes of cardio. You've put yourself in a state similar to that of waking up from a good night's sleep with your glucose depleted. If it's not possible to do it in the morning, then cardio after strength training is the key.

Chapter IX

THE REAL WORK—
RESISTANCE OR STRENGTH TRAINING

Let's go to resistance or strength training. This may be my favorite pastime. You're going to say, "Isn't this just bodybuilding?" My answer? No. Is it absolutely necessary to getting more healthy than you are now? Maybe not. Like I said: eating is 80% of this. If you eat right you'll be a lot more healthy. But to get extra benefits you do the cardio, right? After all, you've seen plenty of programs that ask for some physical exertion, so running, biking, or whatever is no big deal. The cardio adds to that 80%. And once you've gotten that far doesn't it make sense to want to be in the best shape possible, as fast as possible? Of course it does. So if you want to get every health benefit you can from peeling off fat, and if you want to feel better than you ever have, you'll do these exercises too. They are what bring you up to 100%. So I'm going to tell you now: it's necessary.

With that established, I strongly suggest that your cardio and strength training be performed on the same day, 20 minutes of each three-to-four days per week. Choose your days, or simply work out every other day. It matters not. I suggest this because your increased metabolic rate from your new diet and your exercise day will carry completely over through your off day.

Now, let's be frank: is there a bodybuilding component in what I'm about to tell you? Of course there is. Some of you want that more than others. To those of you who don't, I still want the 20 minutes. Try it and see.

To the rest of you: Do I hear you saying you want to be huge and ripped? The only way you'll get there is to lift heavy and hard and eat often. This is my motto.

Strength training has been a big part of my life since middle school. Unfortunately, that was about thirty years ago, but for twenty-five of those years I did strength training without proper nutrition. I have to discount most of that time.

Though I did perfect my technique, form, and performance of most strength training exercises (you can do this in a month), I was far away from achieving my goals because I didn't know how to eat. All those years I kept asking myself why I didn't look like the guys in *Muscle and Fitness* magazine. It's all diet, my friends.

This book can be a help to the bodybuilder, but I'm writing it for the non-athletes among you: those of you who've never touched a plate, dumbbell or barbell. Why? Because we've got to have a baseline. Yes, I'm clearly capable of writing a bodybuilders manual but why should I? These guys already know how to train. If you know how to strength train, all you'll need to learn is how to eat, and I've shown you that.

My biggest goal is to help those who have struggled and lost. As I said before: it is for those at their wits end who are considering a gastric bypass because nothing will work. I love to watch the fat melt away from people like you, and the strength training makes it melt faster.

The *Turning Back the Hands of Time Strength Training System* is based solely on an adjustable bench and a pair of adjustable dumbbells. That's it! That's all you'll need to completely change your life. It will be remarkable.

First: muscle physiology. There are three types of muscle tissue in the body: skeletal, cardiac, and smooth muscle.

Cardiac muscle makes up the heart, and smooth muscle makes up most of our gastrointestinal tract. Cardiac and smooth muscle are involuntarily controlled.

Skeletal muscle is what we're interested in. It's also called striated muscle and is attached to bone via tendons. Usually skeletal muscle is attached to two separate bones across a joint. Contraction of a skeletal muscle causes the muscle to shorten, moving the bones. Hence the purpose (in general) of skeletal muscle is to move the skeleton. Some skeletal muscles between ribs and vertebra have more of a structural component. These don't concern us. Generally skeletal muscle is voluntarily controlled, *i.e.* we control the contraction of the muscle.

Each muscle has an outer covering of connective tissue called the epimysium. When you stretch prior to strength training this is what you are stretching. Our goal behind stretching is to give muscles room to expand. The more we stretch the epimysium, the more room the muscle has to expand. I will give you complete instructions on stretching prior to strength training.

Under the epimysium the muscle tissue is divided into fascicles, which contain up to 150 cells or fibers. Within the fibers, the contractile proteins are grouped into bundles called myofibrils. The contractile proteins themselves are called myofilaments. The proteins within the myofilaments are called Actin and Myosin.

These interact with one another in sort of a ratchet mechanism, which is called a sarcomere.

In general, when we resistance train, we break down the sarcomere and cause inflammation. Bodybuilders know this as Delayed Onset Muscle Soreness (DOMS). With the proper nutrition, *i.e.* Branched Chain Amino Acids (BCAAs) and other amino acids, the muscles repair the damage and build more actin and myosin. This makes the muscles bigger and stronger.

Even before high school I use to see the Charles Atlas ad. It was the one on the back of the comic book where the bully on the beach walked off with the girl after kicking sand in the skinny kid's face. The next year, after the skinny kid had done Mr. Atlas's program, he was back on the beach, all muscles, and getting all the girls. I saved all my grass cutting money and ordered the program. My parents gave me a 110-pound standard set of barbells for my birthday and off I went.

At that time those who studied the science of muscle physiology believed that with weight training the number of muscle cells increased, a process which was called *hyperplasia*. As we learned more about kinesiology, (the science of exercise and muscle physiology) we learned that what really happened was *hypertrophy*, not *hyperplasia*. In other words, the number of contractile proteins within the muscle cell increased, making the cells themselves bigger. God and your parents gave you a finite number of muscle cells. That is the genetics behind bodybuilding and muscle development.

I could get into further scientific intricacies, but for the 99% of you who aren't scientists, suffice to say: the body is an infinitely complex organism. Every move we make requires complicated signals to pass between the brain and the body. What concerns us is how to train our muscles to grow. The essential first step is nutrition. We have to feed the muscles good complex carbohydrates for energy and lean protein for repair. With these they have the potential for growth.

Our goal for resistance training is to increase our lean tissue mass. Skeletal muscle is the most metabolically active tissue in our bodies. The more skeletal muscle we have, the more fat we'll burn. In other words, we want to grow the muscle and let the body burn its own fat.

Skeletal muscle weighs much more than fat, so for many of you burning off fat and gaining muscle tissue will actually bring an overall weight gain. This is one more reason to stay off the scale. Don't worry about weight loss; it's not in our interest. When you begin to body stat and see the lean tissue gain and fat loss you'll know you're on the right track!

We start with stretching. Stretching is required prior to any strength training exercise. It's the way we warm our muscles and our joints prior to placing them under the stress of resistance training. A study by Duke University Medical Center found clearly that stretching prior to exercise significantly reduces the risk of muscle strain.

It's best that you stretch not only prior to resistance training, but between sets and after exercise. Stretching will squeeze out metabolic byproducts which build up in the muscle during exercise. The aim is to make your recovery of that muscle group less painful. Stretching also helps break up adhesion between muscle bundles. This can lead to inflammation and effect repair of muscle protein. Lastly stretching will lengthen or enlarge the facial sheath around the muscle to allow for more muscular growth.

Prior to doing stretching techniques, we should cover the major muscle groups you will be working. You'll see what I mean when we arrive at my split training technique for any given week.

Chest – The chest is mainly made up of the pectoralis major and pectoralis minor muscle, (the pecs).

Back – The latissimus dorsi and rhomboid major are adductors of the arm and shoulder respectively. The trapezius, is an elevator of the shoulder.

Arms – The biceps muscle is a flexor of the arm, and the triceps muscle is an extensor of the arm

Shoulders – The anterior middle and posterior heads of the deltoid make up the shoulder. They rotate and abduct the arm.

Legs – The front of the thigh is made up of the quadriceps muscles. The quads are a group of four muscles: the rectus femorus, vastas lateralis, vastas medialis and the sartorius. All these muscles extend the leg. The back of the thigh is made up of the hamstring muscle. This muscle is made up of the semi-membranous muscle, semi-tendonous muscle and the long and short biceps femoris. The hamstring flexes the lower leg. The calf is an elevator of the heel. The main muscles of the calf are the gastrocnemius and peroneus.

Abdomen – The muscles of the core are the rectus abdominis, which flexes the core, and the lateral oblique, which is an adductor of the core.

Again, the philosophy behind *Turning Back the Hands of Time* is that anything you want can be achieved with a pair of

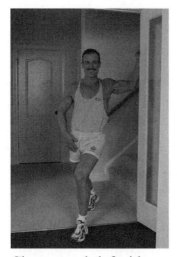

Chest stretch-left side

adjustable dumbbells and an adjustable bench. Period! So, let's get stretching.

There are two ways to stretch the chest: you can use your adjustable bench in the fully upright position, or you can use a door jam. With your elbows bent at almost 90 degrees, place your hand on the door jam, or on the top of the adjustable bench, and step forward, putting pressure on your hand and stretching the pecs. You should feel tension in your chest on the side against which you're leaning. Now, stretch the other side in the same fashion.

When you stretch the back, again you can use your bench or any stationary pole. With the bench in the upright position place yourself behind it. Hold the sides of the upright bench and lean back. Make sure you hold low on the bench so it won't turn over. With your arms completely extended,

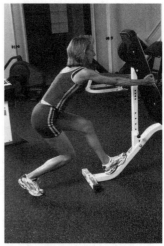

Back stretch

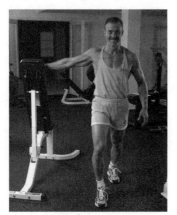

Arm stretch

you are leaning back, and you feel pulling and stretching of the Lats.

When you stretch the arms, you will stretch both the bis and tris. For the biceps, you will use the bench in its upright position. Make a fist, and with your arm out straight at your side, put it against the top of the upright bench. The top, *i.e.* the thumb and index finger portion of the fist should be against the cushion of the bench. As you did with the chest, gently step forward with your leg closest to the bench and feel the stretch in your bicep. To stretch the tricep go to the door jam. Put your back against the door jam and bend your knees. Now reach over your head and

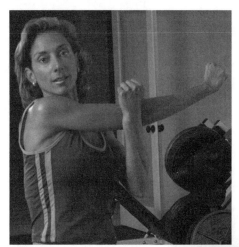

grab the door jam. Hold on tight. Now stand up slowly, but don't let your hands move. Feel the stretch in your tris.

When you stretch your shoulders, you use your body. When stretching the right shoulder, hold your right arm straight out in front of your body.

Shoulder stretch-right

Now, fold it over your chest and capture your straight right arm with your left arm. At about the area of the triceps, pull tight to your body. This will stretch the posterior deltoids. Reverse arms and repeat for the left shoulder. For the anterior and the middle deltoids put your straight

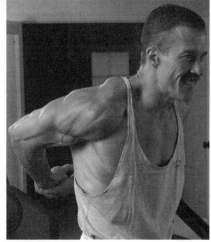

Shoulder stretch

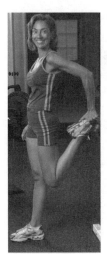

Quadricep

arms behind your back and clasp your fingers. Raise your arms as high as you can. Feel the stretch in your anterior and middle deltoids.

When you stretch your quadriceps, you can use the bench and your hands. First, place the bench at an angle between 30 and 45 degrees. Walk behind the bench, balance yourself and place the top of your foot on the elevated portion of the bench.

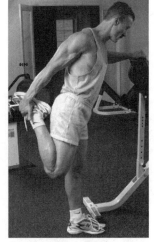

Runner's stretch

Gently lean back. Feel the stretch in your quads. You can also use the runner's stretch. Balance yourself, bend your leg, and grasp the top of your right foot with your right

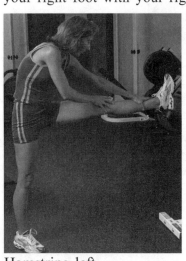

Hamstring-left

hand. Pull your leg up and stretch your quad. Be sure to do both legs with one of these methods.

In stretching the hamstring, place the bench in a flat position. Put your heel on the bench and grasp your leg as low as you can. Lean as far forward as you can while you stretch out your hamstring. Repeat this procedure with the other leg

When stretching the calf you will need a wall. Again this is a runner's stretch. Stand two-to-three feet from the wall.

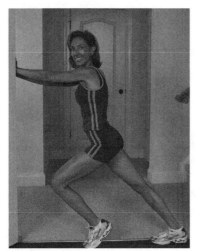

Calf stretch

Put your right foot back. With the sole of your foot on the ground lean forward with both hands on the wall and push back. Feel the stretch in your calf. Now do the other leg.

Finally, let's stretch the abdomen and the obliques. For the abs, simply put your hands over your head or on the back

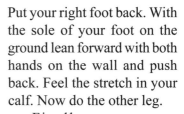

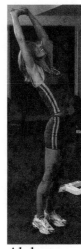

of your head while standing up. Lean back and stretch the abs. When you stretch the left and right obliques, stand and place your right hand on your hip, reach over your head with your left arm   Abdomen

and lean to the right. Lean as far as you can while stretching your left obliques. Now do the other side.

This may seem like a lot of stretching, but now you come to split training where you only work out one or two muscle groups at a time. Therefore you will only have to stretch out one or two groups of muscles per day of exercise.

Obliques   Stretching is done slowly and conservatively. You don't bounce when you stretch! You feel the muscle stretch then hold it for a few seconds to lengthen the muscle fibers and warm them up.

At lectures, people always ask about when to exercise what body parts. They say that they exercise their upper body on one day and their lower body on the other. That's fine if you only exercise twice a week, but I would rather you exercised four times a week.

This is what I was talking about when I said: split training. It's exercising only one or two major muscle groups in a day. You train these muscle groups to failure causing breakdown of the contractile proteins, then rest these muscles for a week, letting them heal, repair, and grow. If you exercise your entire upper body two times per week you are not taking the major muscle groups to failure and you are not allowing them time to heal.

In resistance training you will train in groups of sets. Sets are groups of exercises made up of repetitions. For example, if I lay flat on the bench and press the dumbbells upward ten times, I have done one set of ten reps.

I want you to do twenty minutes of resistance training three-to-four times per week preferably on the same days as your cardio training.

I do one major muscle group each day. If you work out three or four times per week you will need to combine two major muscle groups. If you are very motivated and strength train four times per week for 20 minutes per session, this is what I'd like you to do:

Day 1 – Chest and Arms
Day 2 – Back and Shoulders
Day 3 – Quads and Hams
Day 4 – Abs and Calves

You'll exercise each major muscle group for ten minutes, then you'll move to the next group. In twenty minutes you're done. Don't forget to stretch for five minutes prior to the exercise, and while you are resting between sets.

If you choose to only exercise three times per week you'll have to double up a bit. That's why four times is better; with four times you can spend a good ten minutes on each major muscle group.

It has always been thought that to gain mass you need to do fewer reps, but work out with heavier weights, and to gain tone you should use lighter weights and do more reps. I'm not sure that's true. I've been doing this a long time and I've come to think there's only one way to train with weights: to failure whether you're using light or heavy weights.

Go very light on your first set. This is a warm-up set to get your muscles acclimated to the exercise. After that you can use heavier weights.

It's critical that you never use more weight then you can comfortably handle. Form and range of motion (fully extending and fully contracting) are everything in weight training. Use a comfortable weight. Do your repetitions slowly using excellent form and full range of motion, and take the exercise to failure (i.e. your muscle just can't contract again to do another rep). Then stop and rest. Rest time should be approximately 30 seconds to one minute between sets.

I was recently watching one of those infomercials with claims for an ab machine that was guaranteed to give you perfect form for every rep. They said that with only two minutes of work per day you would have a ripped six-pack. What a crock! One thing we should all realize: there is no such thing as perfect form. If you watch Ronnie Coleman (Mr. Olympia) or Kevin Levrone (multiple top five finisher in the Olympia) do bench presses, you will see that each has his own form. One is no better than the other. Using the basics of good form, each of them has developed a form that is right for him. So, let me repeat: There's no such thing as perfect form. Strive for good form in strength training. Good form with good range of motion, and safe, manageable weight is critical in order to avoid injury. Just do it, and do it safely.

There's a lot of coaching about breathing. Some think that proper form should be inhaling on the eccentric phase (relaxation phase) of the rep and exhaling on the concentric phase (contraction phase) of the rep. In other words, using our flat bench dumbbell press as an example, you should breathe out when you press the dumbbell up and breathe in when you let the dumbbell back down. I believe you should breathe when you need to breathe. Have it be natural. Most of all never hold your breath.

I practice the diamond philosophy of strength training. My first set is light, the tip of the diamond, and I gradually get heavier i.e. the middle of the diamond and then I do one last light set which I call a burnout set, *i.e.* the other tip of the diamond. This burnout set stresses the muscle and breaks down the contractile proteins.

But above all BE CAREFUL! This is serious stuff. You can get hurt. Pay attention. Think about what you're doing at all times. Two years ago I was doing a squat of 505 pounds. For a moment I let my attention wander to the TV. I dropped the bar on my leg and it snapped my fibula like a twig! No training for two months. I was lucky it didn't break both bones in my lower leg. I was also glad that it was off season.

So, let's get started. I'm going to give you multiple exercises for each muscle group. Try them all and change them. Keep it interesting. With the different exercises you can hit the muscle at difficult angles and stimulate faster growth.

CHEST

Flat Bench Dumbbell Press:

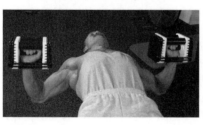

With the bench flat, lie down. Bring the dumbbells to the side of your chest with elbows bent. Push the dumbbells straight up over your chest. Hold them there, then slowly bring them back to starting position. Your palms are facing away from your face during this exercise, and the position of the dumbbell does not change.

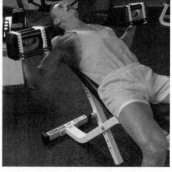

Incline Bench Dumbbell Press & Decline Bench Dumbbell Press:

These are exactly the same with the exception of the angulations of the bench. In both exercises the incline of the bench should be around 30 degrees whether up or down. The flat bench press hits the entire pectoralis muscle while the decline focuses on the lower pectoralis and the incline focuses on the upper pectoralis.

Flat Bench Dumbbell Flies:
    This exercise will be much more difficult than the press, so use much lighter weights. While the bench is flat, lie down and hold the dumbbells over your chest with your palms facing each

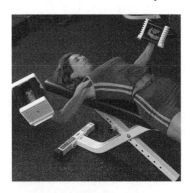

other, and a slight bend to your elbows. Slowly bring the dumbbells out to your side, arms still straight, with a slight bend of the elbows. At the bottom of the rep contract your pecs, and bring the dumbbells back to the top, over your chest. Now repeat the movement.

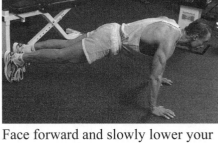

Pushups and Decline Pushups:
    Everyone knows what a pushup is. Done correctly your toes are on the floor, as are your palms, and your body is held up by extended arms. Your hands should be slightly more than shoulder width.

Face forward and slowly lower your chin to the floor. Now push yourself up.
    Decline pushups are exactly the same except your toes are stationed on the bench not the floor. You're on a much more severe angle, putting much greater pressure on your pectoralis muscles.

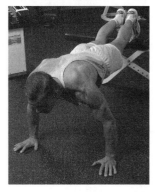

BACK

One-Arm Dumbbell Rows:

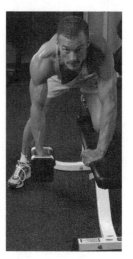

This is one of my favorites. Grasp the dumbbell with your right palm facing inward. Kneel on the bench with your left knee. Bend over and support your upper body with your left hand on the bench. Pull your right hand directly upward, keeping your elbow close to your body. Stop when the dumbbell gets to your stomach height, then slowly lower it.

Dumbbell Dead Lifts:

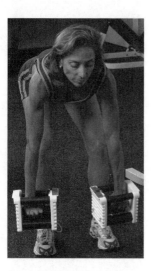

Be careful with this exercise because your back is in jeopardy. Use very light weights to start to get your form down. Place the dumbbells on the floor. Bend at the knees and waist. KEEP YOUR BACK STRAIGHT and your butt out and back. Look up and forward. The dumbbells are grasped either with palms facing backward or inward. Slowly stand straight up keeping your arms straight. Now slowly lower yourself back down, but don't lay the dumbbells on the ground. Repeat the motion.

Dumbbell Bent Over Rows:

Again your back is important here so pay attention to form, and use light weights until you get your form down. Grasp the dumbbells again with palms facing inward or backward. Back straight and your butt is back. Look forward. From your straight arm position pull the dumbbells straight up to your chest. If your palms are inward, keep your elbows close to your body when you lift the dumbbells.

Dumbbell Shrugs:

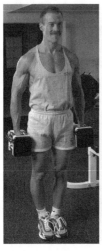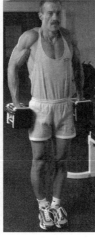

This exercise works the trapezius muscle. Stand straight up with the dumbbells at your sides palms facing inward. Simply shrug your shoulders straight up as high as you can. Hold it, then let the weights down slowly to starting position.

BICEPS

Alternating Dumbbell Curls:

Standing straight up hold the dumbbells at your sides with palms facing inward. Elevate one dumbbell at a time by bending your elbow. Bring the dumbbell up as high as you can and rotate the palms upward during the concentric phase of the exercise. Return the dumbbell to its starting position.

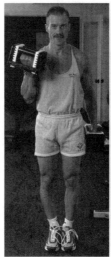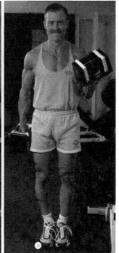

Simultaneous Dumbbell Curls:

These are basically the same as the alternating dumbbell curls, except you elevate both dumbbells at the same time. These can either be done with the rotating motion or from start to finish; the palms can be facing forward.

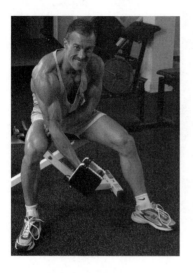

Concentration Curls:

Sitting on the flat bench spread your knees apart. Hold the dumbbell in your right hand and rest your right elbow on the innermost part of your right thigh. Support your elbow with your left hand. Your left elbow is resting on your left thigh. Bend over slightly and lower the dumbbell between your legs with your right hand, then curl it back up to the starting position.

Incline Dumbbell Curls:

This is a killer. Incline the bench to about 30 degrees. Sit on the bench and hold one dumbbell in each hand straight down from your shoulder palms facing forward. Curl each dumbbell up alternating or together.

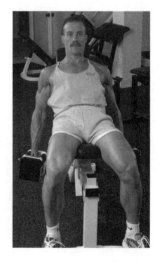

21s: Another killer! While standing, hold the dumbbells at your sides, your palms facing forward. Curl the dumbbells together to the position of your waist for seven reps. Next curl the dumbbells from your waist to your chest for seven reps. Now curl the dumbbells all the way from your side to your chest for seven reps. All twenty-one reps are done at once without rest.

TRICEPS

Dumbbell Kickbacks:
Assume the same position on the bench as if you were doing dumbbell rows for your back. Hold the dumbbell with your right

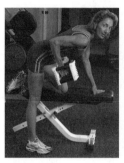 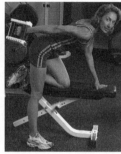

hand palm facing inward. Your right elbow is kept at your side and your arm is kept at a 90-degree angle. Now straighten your elbow, moving the dumbbell in a backward direction until your arm is straight. Return the dumbbell to the starting position.

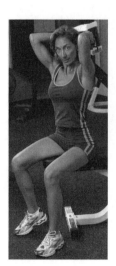

Dumbbell Overhead Presses:
Sit on the flat bench and grasp a dumbbell with your palms facing up and in under the top of the dumbbell. Don't grasp the handle of the dumbbell. Hold the dumbbell

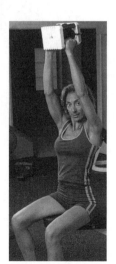

directly over your head, with your elbows by your ears. Slowly lower the dumbbell behind your head to the level of your shoulders. Always keeping your elbows inward, raise the dumbbell back up to its starting position.

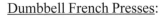

Dumbbell French Presses:

Holding the dumb-bell just as you did on the last exercise, lay flat on the bench looking upward. Hold the dumbbell at arms' length over your head and face. While keeping your elbows in, lower the dumbbell until it nearly touches your forehead. Keep your elbows in, and push the dumbbell directly back upward to the starting position.

Tricep Pushups:

Elevate the bench to its highest position. Stand behind the bench and place your hands on the back of the upright. Now move your feet well away from the bench. Lean all the way forward while bending your arms and supporting your body weight until your forehead nearly touches your hand. Keeping your elbows as close as you can, push your body back to its starting position.

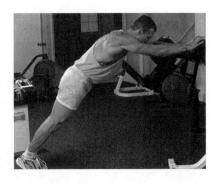

SHOULDERS

Dumbbell Military Press:

There are many variations of this exercise. It can be done standing or seated. Your palms can be inward or facing forward. With this exercise mix it up, as different variations will hit different areas of the deltoid muscle. While seated hold the dumbbells at head level. Push the dumbbells directly upward until your arms

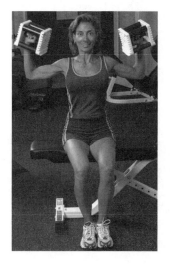

are fully extended. Now return the dumbbells to the starting position. Again, change your palm position from time to time. You can either alternate the reps or do them simultaneously.

Arnold Dumbbell Presses:

This is a simple variation of the military press. While seated or standing hold the dumbbells at ear level with your palms facing inward. Raise the dumbbells as you rotate your palm forward during the rep. After full extension lower the dumbbells to their starting position.

Inclined Dumbbell Shoulder Press:

This is a variation on the military press. Simply incline the bench to a 45-degree angle. Lay on the bench. Dumbbells are at the level of your ears. Push directly upward. Vary your palm position and do reps simultaneously or alternating.

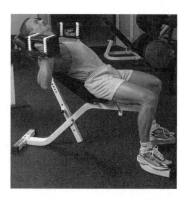

Dumbbell Flies:

Dumbbell flies can be done either to the front or the sides. To the side, hold the dumbbell with your palms facing inward. Slowly elevate the dumbbells to your sides until your arms are straight out and parallel to the floor. Lower the dumbbells.

To the front, start with your palms facing backward. Elevate your dumbbells forward until your arms are parallel with the floor. Now back to the starting position.

Dumbbell Rows:

This is one of the best upper body exercises out there. Stand with your feet spread to the width of your shoulders. Hold the dumbbell handle with both hands down around your thighs in front of your body. Keeping the dumbbell close to your body, lift it in one motion, with both hands, to around your chin. Elbows are obviously straight out at your sides during this

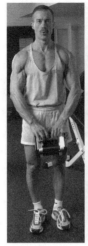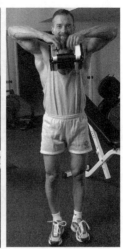

exercise. Slowly return the dumbbell to its starting position.

ABDOMEN

I don't overemphasize abdomen exercises. A lot of trainers do and I don't know why. Your abs are no different than any other major muscle group. Why work them differently? If anything, I work them less because these are my least favorite exercises.

Remember: you will never, and I mean never, have a ripped six-pack abdomen because of resistance training. A ripped abdomen is a product of cardiovascular training and your *Hands of Time* nutrition plan. So if you want to get that six-pack do these exercises to tone the abs but get on your cardio and eat clean!

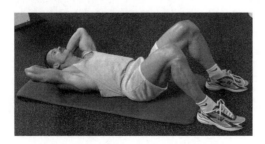

Floor Crunches:

Have a mat or at least a towel to lie on. Lie on the floor with your knees bent and soles flat on the ground. Place your

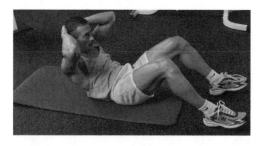

hands behind your head, and lean forward, lifting up at the abdomen, bringing your nose toward your knees. Feel the stomach muscles tighten and burn. Now return to your starting position. This is not a sit-up. You're not sitting all the way up. You are simply crunching forward then back to start.

Crunches with Legs Elevated:

This is exactly the same exercise but this time we're going to place our calf muscles on the flat bench then crunch upwards.

Either of these crunches can be done while holding a weight of some sort behind your head.

Bench Abdominal Crunches:

This is a tough exercise and will take some getting used to. Sit on the flat bench as you would if you were going to straddle it. Put your hands behind your back, around your butt to stabilize yourself. Bring your knees up. While stabilizing yourself lean back, and at the same time straighten your legs out a bit. Crunch forward trying to bring your knees and nose together. Now back to starting position.

Leg Raises:

Leg raises are simply that—raising your legs and holding them there. This can be done on the bench or floor. It may be a little easier on the bench. Place the bench at a 30-degree angle, lie back and support your balance with your hands on the bench under your butt. Elevate your legs to a 30-degree angle and hold them there. When I do this I sometimes spread them and bring them back together just to kill time. Then I put them back down to rest. Don't rest too long because that was only one repetition. Do it again.

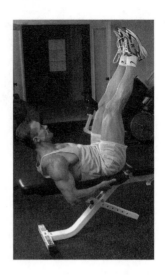

CALVES

There are a couple of really good exercises for the calf muscles. Both involve a stairwell.

Two-Legged Calf Raise:

While in the stairwell balance yourself against the wall. Place your toes and the balls of your feet on the stair, but let the rest of your foot extend out off the step. Slowly lower yourself down and allow your foot to flex as your heel gets closer to the next step down. Now extend your toes as much as possible as if you were trying to stand on your toes. Do it again.

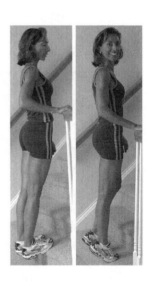

One-Leg Calf Raise:

This is exactly the same exercise but you're only standing on one leg. Rest your other foot around the heel of the foot that's working. Slowly lower yourself and raise yourself as was previously described. Remember, this will be more difficult than the two-leg calf raise because all of your weight will be on that one calf muscle.

HAMSTRINGS

Straight Leg Dumbbell Deadlifts:

This is another exercise where you want to watch your back. Go very lightweight until you understand the form and the range

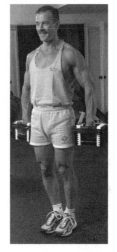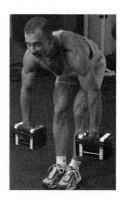

of motion of the exercise. Hold the dumbbells at your sides with palms facing backward. With only the slightest bend of your knees, bend down, keeping your back straight, head up and butt back. Lower the dumbbells almost to the ground or as low as you can carefully go. Now stand directly up again, with only the slightest bend of the knee, feeling the burn and stretching of the hamstring.

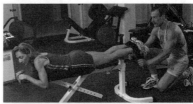
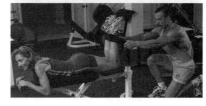

Bench Hamstring Curls:

This is the only exercise here that will take some assistance from a helper. Lay face down on the bench. Keep your knees close together, so when your legs are extended they are hanging off the bench. Extend your knees and have your partner place a towel over your ankles. Now have that person hold resistance on the dangling portion of the towel while you flex your hamstring and curl your legs up. As you return to starting position your partner should continue to hold tension on the towel to create work on the muscle both eccentrically and concentrically

QUADRICEPS

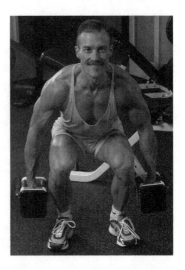

Dumbbell Squats:

This is exactly what it sounds like. You stand and hold the dumbbells at your waist, palms inward. Your feet are about shoulder-width apart. Very slowly you squat down, not too low, but low enough that when you return to standing position you feel the quad working. Make sure to keep your back straight at all times here.

Dumbbell Lunges:

Lunges are excellent exercises. They can be done either in a standing position or while walking. With a lunge you hold the dumbbells at your side. Then you lunge out with one leg or the

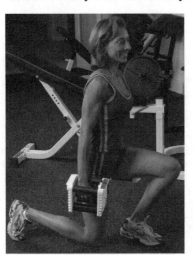

other. If you lunge out or step forward with the right leg, the left foot stays stationary, but the knee of the left leg in particular goes forward and down close to the floor. Then push back with your right leg to the starting position and lunge forward with the left leg. I prefer walking lunges, but my wife likes stationary. They are equally as beneficial for the quadriceps.

Dumbbell Step Ups:

This exercise begins with dumbbells at your sides, palms facing inward. You are standing in front of the bench. Being careful not to lose your balance, lift your right leg and step up on the bench bringing your left foot up until you are standing on the bench. Now step back and off of the bench with your left leg first, and your right leg follows you down. Now repeat this exercise by stepping up with the left foot.

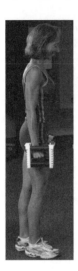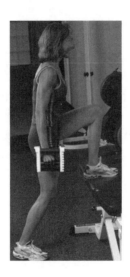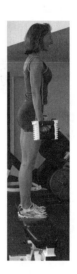

In a nutshell, you've learned all the dumbbell exercises it will take to get you into the best health and shape of your life. My gut feeling is that you will start to enjoy this so much that you'll spend more then twenty minutes at it. But believe me if you follow my nutrition plan and do this, along with twenty minutes of cardiovascular exercises three-to-four times per week on the same day, the changes should be astronomical.

It's never too late to start strength training. You can start at any age and gain benefit. An article in a recent nutrition periodical stated the average male over forty years old will lose on average ten pounds of lean mass and gain fifteen pounds of fat every ten years. With my plan, you will lose no mass and will gain no fat. Strength training stimulates the skeletal muscles and with the proper nutrition your goal will be to gain more lean mass and cut off all the fat. Don't let yourself be part of that statistic.

And to the elderly: Have you ever noticed how elderly people are more immobile than the rest of us. If this isn't rheumatoid arthritis or degenerative joint disease, it is probably simple disuse. As we get older we do less. Our muscles, joints and bones become stiffer and less functional. One way that elderly people can maintain function and mobility of the muscles and joints is by strength training.

What about women over forty? You may be the ones who need resistance training the most. With the lack of estrogen in post-menopausal women, bone density decreases and osteoporosis can set in. In other words, the bones get brittle. Study after study shows that resistance training not only stimulates muscle tissue, but also stimulates an increase in bone density, and can reverse or halt the progression of osteoporosis.

Chapter X

TURNING BACK THE HANDS OF TIME

In conclusion, I'd like to thank you for spending your valuable time reading this book. I hope you've learned more about your health and physique.

I've given you a lot of information; it's all tried and true. I promise it will work. The nutrition portion of the book is the most important. As you heard me say time and time again, you are what you eat. It's 80 % nutrition. For real!

If you follow my diet to the letter and do no cardio and no resistance training at all, you will lose a ton of fat, but the process will be very slow, and you won't be toned and firm. By stimulating our metabolic rates with cardiovascular exercises and building and toning more skeletal muscle, we actually turn our bodies into fat-burning machines.

I hope you fall in love with this lifestyle, becoming so addicted to it that you say: "The hell with this Emmett guy, I'm doing thirty minutes of cardio and an hour of strength training five days a week!" I hope I hear you telling anyone who wants to hear: "This egg white omelet with veggies is really good, and by the way, I'm sure looking forward to that Martini, standing rib roast and chocolate cake on Saturday night!" When a friend asks how you got so fit, I want you to start by saying: "I'm eating more food than I've ever eaten in my entire life."

One very important cautionary note: You absolutely MUST consult your internist or family practice doctor prior to initiating my program. If you have uncontrolled heart disease, kidney disease or diabetes, this plan may not be right for you. Listen to your doctor and follow his or her advice. As long as you're walking, talking, and breathing, your doctor will almost certainly give you the green light. After all, they might want to counterbalance that colleague of theirs who told us to eat a pound of bacon for breakfast because it was carbohydrate-free.

❈ ❈ ❈

Baltimore's a small town—a two-person town, they say. In a two-person town if you don't know someone, at least you know someone who knows them. So, in the fall of 2002 there was quite a stir when several big time local amateur athletes—bikers, marathoners and such—all members of the medical community—dropped dead for no apparent reason. Two were out enjoying their sports when they fell; others were at home. Death took them, all within a few weeks. It shook our community. One of them was my best friend.

Shortly after, I spoke to a cardiologist friend. She told me, "John, it's not the diagnosed cardiovascular disease that will get you. It's the one you don't know about." So, again, by all means, have an exam, an EKG, a stress test or an echo if your MD suggests. Follow your doctor's directions.

Remember, I'm here to help make you healthy, but again this is a huge lifestyle change. It's one that will work! Now that I've given you the knowledge, you have to get off your butt and find the discipline and incentive within yourself to finish the job. Trust me. Believe me and follow my directive, and you will truly change your life once and for all. Thank you for allowing me to help you TURN BACK THE HANDS OF TIME.

ABOUT THE AUTHOR

Dr. John Emmett was born in Toledo, Ohio. In 1972, his family settled in Baltimore, Maryland. He attended Randolph Macon College, followed by a year of post-graduate studies at the College of William & Mary.

Dr. Emmett returned to Baltimore to study at the University of Maryland Dental School, graduating in 1989. After a year with the Veterans Administration in a General Practice Residency, he trained in Oral and Maxillofacial Surgery at the Georgetown University Medical Center, and then established a solo practice at the Saint Joseph Medical Center. Dr. Emmett is the recipient of numerous professional awards and honors.

An avid athlete throughout his life, he is active as a youth sports' coach for multiple recreation councils. Strength training or lifting weights have always been a major part of Dr. Emmett's philosophy and practice. Around the same time he began amateur competitive bodybuilding, he recognized.the importance of nutrition in his overall plan. Since then, using the "Hands of Time" nutrition and exercise program, he has attained the following championship titles:

- 2004 NPC Mr. Maryland Masters Champion
- 2004 NABBA Maryland State Cup Overall Champion
- 2004 USBF Maryland Silver Cup Masters Champion
- 2003 USBF Maryland Silver Cup Masters Champion
- 2003 USBF Baltimore Natural Pro-Am Masters Champion
- 2003 USBF York Pennsylvania Natural Light Heavyweight Champion
- 2003 USBF York Pennsylvania Natural Masters Champion
- 2002 NABBA Maryland State Cup Light Heavyweight Champion
- 2002 NABBA Maryland State Cup Masters Champion

He lives in Phoenix, Maryland with his wife, Dr. Margie Hernandez, a pediatric dentist and body builder, and their two children, John and Alexis.

For more information, please consult our website:

www.nufitness.net